THE YOUTH CORRIDOR

THE YOUTH CORRIDOR

A Renowned Plastic Surgeon's Revolutionary Program for Maintenance, Rejuvenation, and Timeless Beauty

GERALD IMBER, M.D.

WILLIAM MORROW AND COMPANY, INC.
NEW YORK

It is the policy of William Morrow and Company, Inc., and its imprints and affiliates, recognizing the importance of preserving what has been written, to print the books we publish on acid-free paper, and we exert our best efforts to that end.

Library of Congress Cataloging-in-Publication Data

Imber, Gerald.
The youth corridor : a renowned plastic surgeon's revolutionary program for maintenance, rejuvenation, and timeless beauty / Gerald Imber. — 1st ed.
p.   cm.
ISBN 0–688–14936–7
1. Skin—Care and hygiene.   2. Skin—Aging.   3. Beauty, Personal.
RL 87.I457   1997
646.7'26—DC20   96-24079
                                        CIP

Printed in the United States of America

First Edition

1 2 3 4 5 6 7 8 9 10

BOOK DESIGN BY KAY SCHUCKHART

"... for mothers and fathers,
sons and lovers ..."

ACKNOWLEDGMENTS

Support and encouragement are essential for an individual to pursue this sort of project, particularly as its demands draw time from the other pursuits of life. Therefore, I must first thank Cathryn Collins, who is convinced that the first light of day comes from the word processor, and who secretly enjoyed my absences for the peace and quiet.

The idea of this book was little more than talk until Michael Gross encouraged me to get to it and introduced me to my agent, Elizabeth Kaplan, who liked the idea and helped it find its way to Claire Wachtel at William Morrow. Claire immediately got the point, and was intelligent, helpful, encouraging, and professional throughout. Suzie Derienzo helped pore through the medical literature, Myrna Laureano copied, printed and reprinted, and continually bailed me out of computer trouble. Katie Langer, as usual, ran my life when I was otherwise engaged. My sons, Greg, Jason, and Peter, were always available to retrieve text from the ether. For that, and their constant interest, I thank them. And last, Cisco, who doggedly rose with me each morning, didn't complain about the cigars and the cussing, and remains my loyal friend.

Most of all, my thanks to the classroom of life, where one learns more than one teaches.

G.I.

CONTENTS

PREFACE

~~~~~~~~~~

Most new concepts struggle to see the light of day, until some moment when knowledge and interest begin to fuel one another and the idea takes on a life of its own. Then, everything seems so simple and self-evident that one wonders why it took so long to reach this point. The idea of the Youth Corridor is exactly such a situation. The information was there, the interest was there, but we never put it all together. The purpose of this book is to do just that: condense those bits of information floating about us into an organized, understandable program for controlling aging and maintaining youthful good looks throughout adult life.

The fund of knowledge on aging has enlarged proportionally to our increased life span. Interest in maintaining youthful good looks throughout these expanded years of strength and productivity has run a parallel course. Fueled by fact and fiction, our knowledge has accelerated rapidly and directly through the last decade. I have both participated in and observed this regularly from my perch as a plastic surgeon with an active Manhattan practice, and from the very outset of my professional life I have been consumed by the subject of facial aging. Thousands of face-lifts later I am convinced the tools exist to allow us to deal with the problem in a wholly more appropriate and effective manner. My philosophy, one that has not been universally shared, advocates preventing wrinkles, rather than curing them, and smaller procedures and earlier surgery for generally younger patients, in order to maintain one's appearance throughout the adult years in what I call the Youth Corridor.

Recent advances in biochemistry and new operative techniques have delivered us to a point where our system can forestall, if not prevent, the changes of aging, and push back the need for surgery. We can best provide this service for those who are lucky enough to start caring for themselves before the mirror screams out warnings. For others, we will reset the clock to a new starting point, and help control the future, and in all cases, help you help yourself. This program offers the first organized system incorporating all the latest knowledge to help you live agelessly in the Youth Corridor.

THE YOUTH CORRIDOR

INTRODUCTION

"I was always happy with myself, I looked great. I never thought about changing anything. Sure, there were some signs of aging, but it wasn't terrible. Then, one morning I looked in the mirror, and saw my mother. That was it. I love my mother, but I don't want to look like her. She's a much older woman . . . you know, a different generation, with different priorities. . . ."

There you have it. Given some individual variation in disclaimers, you have the thrust of a story I've heard, on a daily basis, for more than twenty years.

"When did all this happen? What do I do now?"

That question, and the frustration that accompanies it, provide much of the impetus for this book. For anyone who reads fashion magazines, or discusses the subject with friends, the bottom line is simple: Once the damage has been done, nothing short of surgery can restore what has been lost. And even then, the ravages of time cannot be fully undone. Worst of all, so many good years have been spent helplessly watching the changes add up, instead of fighting back. It's frustrating, it's annoying, and yet we simply write it off as the legacy of genetics and the effect of time. There seems nothing worth doing but grind our teeth and wait for things to get worse. But is that really true?

It seemed to me that there had to be a better strategy than watching the horse leave the barn before closing the door. But what to do. I was fully aware of the problem; and the solutions, such as they were, were purely surgical, and aimed at correcting accumulated damage. A case of too much, too late. Or perhaps of appropriate therapy for the stage of aging confronted. Ideally, we would like to alter the speed at which these changes occur, if not prevent them completely. The concept of controlling the signs of aging, if not the process itself, became an issue to which I have devoted a great deal of my professional interest and energies. Some years ago, when I first began to question the conventional approach, I was particularly struck by the absence of treatment options for early changes in younger people, and by the attitude among colleagues that these early changes weren't worth dealing with. It made no sense. If we were going to influence the eventual outcome, the earlier we become involved the better. Attention must be paid to caring for and preventing the earliest signs of aging, preventing wrinkles, not just to curing them, and not solely to reversing the established signs of middle age. Couldn't we rearrange the way we apply our knowledge to the problems of aging? Couldn't we use what we know of anatomy, surgery, medicine, and the chemistry of skin care to help maintain vigorous, good looks, instead of sitting around helplessly watching youthfulness slip away?

Those were pretty much my driving thoughts as I altered and reorganized my priorities within my very traditional practice of plastic surgery. How wonderful if people could maintain their youthful appearance throughout adulthood and middle age. Quality of life counts, and when one has reached a stage of confidence and achievement, why not welcome it looking as good as you feel? We are physically able to maintain an attractive, and naturally youthful, countenance for decades. It is simply a matter of caring enough to make the effort. The information is all available, but organizing it in a manner that makes sense as a helpful program requires understanding of the changes brought on by the years, and a willingness to apply the programs to every stage of adult life. You can look great throughout your adult life. Helping you do so is the problem I have set out to solve.

The book you are about to read may actually change your life. It is the result of the newest advances in the control of facial aging, organized so that you can understand it all, and presented in a fashion applicable to any age. The method will help maintain the youthful good looks of the twenty-five-year-old from today into the future, will stabilize the thirty-five-year-old, offer maintenance and effective options for reversing signs of aging in the forty-five-year-old, and tell the fifty-five-year-old how to reset the clock and keep looking her best. Whatever your age, this information can help you look your best.

Obviously, the best time to begin maintenance is before the changes have begun. Those with enough insight to begin so very early are the lucky few; the rest of us must slow the process, undo the visible changes, and pay more attention to ourselves. There is so much to be learned. Simply eliminating negative influences is an important step in the right direction. If you come away from this book with new insight and an enlightened attitude, you will be on the road to helping yourself. Adopt the program at any stage of life, and you will truly do some good. The deeper you immerse yourself in the routine, the maintenance process, and the applicable procedures, the better you will look. It's as simple as that.

the youth CORRIDOR

what it means and why it is important for you

Much energy has been lavished on the problem of facial aging, and a great deal has changed over the last ten years. If we haven't truly overcome the problem, we have certainly made great progress in our approach and our thinking. The key lies in dealing with the control of the predictable changes—and they are predictable—instead of relying solely on cosmetic surgery after the fact. Not only does this make great sense, it is also applicable to a far wider universe and brings us closer to our goal of living gracefully in the Youth Corridor.

The art and science of plastic surgery arose from the hospital wards of the First World War. It has come far, and changed considerably along the way. We plastic surgeons have been specifically trained to undo damage inflicted upon the human body by genetic accidents, the assault of war, or the slow ravages of time. Ours has not been a world of prevention, and so our thinking has always been skewed toward the big change, the transformation. The world of antiaging surgery is no exception. The big change, the transformation, prevails here as well. Enter the consulting room old and wrinkled, and leave the operating suite rejuvenated. That is how we all think of plastic surgery, or at least how we thought in the past. I am as guilty of this telescopic blindness as you. Perhaps more so. For I, at least, had the benefit of knowing the facts. But, what if we could push the need for that day of transformation ahead, and manage aging with self-help, maintenance, minimal intervention, and small changes. For most people transformations would be become unnecessary, and so many good years would be enjoyed beautifully.

The concept of the Youth Corridor germinated from the seed of this idea. It means, simply, an extended period of years through which one might maintain a thoroughly youthful appearance. An appearance at once at peace with, and appropriate to, the general well-being and success of those very important years from thirty to fifty-five, and beyond. Why fifty-five and not sixty or sixty-five? Simply because that twenty-five-year period is one in which physical changes can be best managed and controlled. The aging of later years presents deeper and greater manifestations, which though they can be helped and relieved, make it unreasonable to expect complete control. During those twenty-five years much can be done to keep one virtually unchanged. That is the Youth Corridor.

The plan for maintenance has evolved successfully through bits and pieces and thousands of patients over a number of years. This book will explain it all to you. But take warning! Don't expect a generalized do-it-yourself book, or some New Age paean to positive thinking, though much of both is actually a part of the plan. There is a great deal you can do for yourself, much you can do with a bit of professional help, and some that is purely the result of professional help. You can accept or reject its elements as you wish. Even the simplest bits of reeducation will have a positive yield, but what you get out is based on what you put in. This is reality, and if you want to keep on looking the way you envision yourself, pay attention. In our dream world the doctor, in a crisp white coat, hands you the steaming beaker and with a benevolent smile says, "Now, drink this and stay young forever!"

Forget it. That's a dream. What you are about to learn is the furthest thing from wishful thinking, but it's real, it works, and no other approach I've heard of is half as good. Not quite a promise in a pot, it does incorporate self-help, and the cosmetic approach wherever honest, effective, and applicable. In fact, much of what can be done consists of minor lifestyle changes and new maintenance routines. The basis for what we will explore together is scientific. I may take some liberties of simplification in order to avoid reinventing the wheel, but I intend to tell it like it is, and it's all about aging. Aging, not beauty, although the two are often carelessly confused. Let us clear that up right away. One person's vision of beauty is often shockingly different from another's, particularly across cultural boundaries. But those boundaries are dissolving as electrons bounce off satellites, and the rush of jet engines cover the globe, and sameness unfortunately begins to prevail.

Beauty takes many forms. Among the Nuba tribes of the Sudan, decorative scarring of the skin is considered an intrinsic ingredient of beauty. Distortion of the lower lip with the insertion of increasingly large hockey-puck-like objects is a crucial element among a largely primitive tribe in the Brazilian rain forest. But, is that very different from the tattoos affected by so many fashion models? Or nose rings, or navel rings, or for that matter, earrings? Beauty is a subjective and culture-dependent issue, whose sphere enlarges, but is, for a while at least, denied universality by the happy fact that we are not a homogeneous planet. Parents here in America very often consider plastic surgery for their children with protruding "cup" ears. Their reasons are quite understandable. Children are merciless in their taunts for deviations from the norm, and parents are responding sensitively to

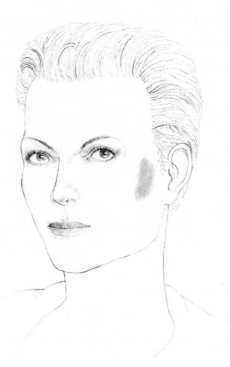

This youthful adult face will be our starting point and our goal.

their children's discomfort. However, in certain counties of Ireland, a majority of the native population boast protruding ears, and are as handsome and normal as can be. Beauty is variable. Aging is an entirely different matter.

Though many cultures genuinely revere the elderly, it is as a group held apart from the bulk of active society. In Western culture our productive years far outstrip our welcome. It's a simple observation of our society. Even the most vain among us grudgingly concede that there is a time to acknowledge age and let nature take its course. But not yet! Not while I'm still young! Not while there is so much to do. That is what we are talking about. Maintaining your youth, not watching it slip away while you pull at your skin and wish things were different. Americans are no longer old at forty, fifty, sixty, or even seventy, and the concept of retiring from a profession or responsible job at sixty-five is a senseless waste of an experienced natural resource. Often, feeling good is directly related to looking good, and the impression we make is how we are perceived. The two go hand in hand. Those who look old and act old are treated differently than those who carry the years well. The average life span for American males is seventy-two years; for females, seventy-nine years. And these are averages. The economically and socially advantaged among us can expect to live far longer. We have learned some of the lessons of medicine, and live generally healthier lives. Science has controlled the potentially lethal afflictions of the first half of the century, and with the advent of antibiotics, medicine has progressed from a science of observation and diagnosis, to one of active intervention and cure. From that point in time to this, the advances have been too fast and furious to list. Happily, as the fortunate beneficiaries, we have assimilated the new order of things, and now take it for granted as our birthright. That's the good news. We can anticipate, and expect to enjoy, unprecedented longevity. As this new reality becomes routine, our focus naturally shifts from survival to quality of life. Diet, exercise, and fashion, and indeed, even cosmetic surgery, have become accepted elements of modern life. We want to look good, and we want it for as long as possible. Though I am a firm believer in the idea of graceful aging, it seems patently ridiculous for people in their forties, fifties, or sixties to tolerate an unnecessarily sagging, wrinkled, aged face. To look old, beaten, and devitalized, when one is anything but that, makes no sense at all.

We will all age in a basically similar manner, even if the outward signs differ. Some of us suffer fine lines and wrinkles as early as our thirties. Others see only a minor loosening of the jawline at fifty. As you will understand, these are all manifestations of the same process. The objective is to keep these signs at bay, not allow them a foothold. When that is not possible, we must stop them in their tracks, before the sum total is a picture of a vital young person trapped in old, ill-fitting skin.

The next chapter will explain how skin ages. We will identify specific trouble areas, show you how to spot your own potential problems, and teach you how to stop them. You will learn an effective skin care routine and a maintenance schedule that can keep you happily within the Youth Corridor, even as your contemporaries grow old around you. If you are lucky enough to begin fighting the battle while you are young, the results will be that much more dramatic, and that much longer lasting.

THREE

fast FORWARD

what
the
years
bring

To fully understand the Youth Corridor, you must first have a general understanding of how we age. The subject is not nearly as terrifying as it sounds, and I'll try to keep the scientific mumbo jumbo to a minimum. After reading these chapters, you will be able to accurately predict how various people will age, and actually pinpoint what action should be taken in various cases. Truly, you will look at strangers in the street, recognize their problems, and know what they must do to stay in the Youth Corridor.

Confining the discussion in this chapter to the skin and its structures

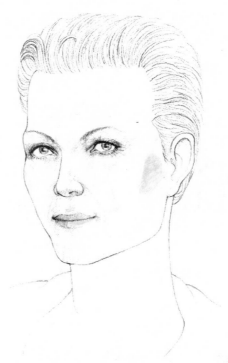

By age thirty-five the first significant changes are visible.

will keep the information from wandering too far afield. However, we must always be mindful of the enormous impact of systemic good health, and certainly systemic illness, on the aging process and, therefore, on one's appearance. A deficiency of the hormone insulin, manufactured in the pancreas, is known to all as the cause of the metabolic disease, diabetes. Sugar intolerance is synonymous with diabetes, and numerous other aspects of the disease are well documented and commonly understood. But diabetes is also associated with impaired small-vessel blood flow. That, too, is well known to the medical community. This may affect various organs over the years. Perhaps the least threatening example of the problem is found in the small blood vessels nourishing the skin. For our purposes, this illustrates an important point. Reduced blood flow through the small vessels of the skin results in reduced nutrient supply and impaired removal of metabolic wastes, and contributes to loss of elasticity, thinning, and oxidation of the collagen layer and wrinkling. Simply put, diabetes causes excessive and early aging of the skin. Is this the most worrisome effect of the disease? Certainly not, but for our purposes it illustrates how important the overall state of health is in determining how one's skin will fare over the years. This knowledge is very fertile ground, and will change the way we think about aging and how we deal with it in the future. But for now we must apply today's solutions to today's problems.

There is no precise point in time when the wear and tear of life begins to take a visible toll on the skin, but there is usually some evidence of change in most people by their thirties. If you are shaking your head in disbelief, think again, look again. Those little squint lines, or smile lines, or whatever acceptable euphemism you choose to hang on them, suddenly surface at about that time. So does the little horizontal line of loose skin under the eyes, and the ever so slight fold of extra skin of the upper lid. "Not so bad," you say. And right you are. But that's the first sign. From here on, the process quickens. Soon the smile lines are deeper and more numerous. They no longer disappear after the smile ends, and they actually seem longer and no longer pleasant. The skin of the upper lid continues to stretch, and begins to look puffy even when you are well rested and living virtuously. It might even be more difficult to apply eye makeup smoothly. Thirty-five, thirty-eight, or maybe forty, but the process has moved along. It started earlier, much earlier, and if we had been more knowledgeable, there is much that could have been done to keep the process under control.

First, you *must* accept that the natural deterioration of the skin begins in your twenties, when the outward signs are absent and you still look great. At this point, your efforts to deal with the process will bear fruit for a future that you haven't yet considered. Many of you are farther down the road, but your own starting point is of less importance than the act of starting itself. At any point of intervention, you will ultimately be better off than if you hadn't started at all. Therefore, this program is for everyone. What is most important is that you want to continue feeling good about yourself, and unless you live in a vacuum, you will agree that looking good plays a major role in that feeling.

how IT HAPPENS

Think of the skin as a form-fitting garment, like tights. They hug your body, move when you move, and as you move. After exposure to the elements, multiple washings, and thousands of bends and folds, the tights begin to sag at the joints and generally loosen all over. That was a description of how your tights age; it's worse for your skin.

Human skin is only fifteen to twenty one thousandths of an inch thick. Thinner than most fabrics. And there is a lot of it, about twenty square feet, which weighs eight to ten pounds. The skin is not just dressing. It is an important functioning organ, made up of two distinct

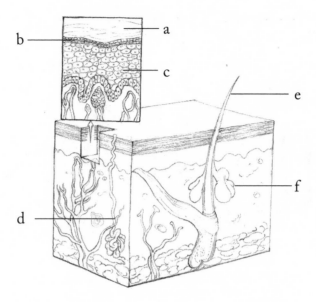

The schematic drawing represents a cross section through human skin.

    a. epidermis
    b. basal layer
    c. dermis
    d. sweat gland
    e. hair
    f. sebaceous (oil) gland

layers called the dermis and the epidermis. The dermis, the deeper of the two lay-ers, is the connection between the skin and the internal body structures. It relates not only to the fat on which the skin rests, or the muscle below, but to the heart, lungs, liver, and the distant endocrine glands, which secrete hormones and regu-late body functions. That is so because the dermis contains the blood vessels that nourish the skin, the nerves that transmit sensations back to the brain, and, in its deepest reaches, the sweat and oil glands of the skin. The substance within which all these important elements reside is largely collagen. Ah, the magic word. Magic, indeed, for it is the state of this collagen that determines the elastic fit of the skin and the presence or absence of wrinkles. Collagen is a protein. A string of amino acids, or small chemical groups, bound to other amino acids. These protein chains are fiberlike, and organized with their neighbors in a regular and predictable pattern. When the pattern is disrupted, broken down, or interfered with, wrinkles result. This collagen damage can occur by repeated actions such as squinting, smiling, or pursing the lips, not at all dissimilar to repeatedly folding and unfolding a piece of paper until it is permanently scored. That is one way a wrinkle forms.

Within the collagen substance is a similar, and related, fiber called elastin. These fibers are responsible for the resilience and elasticity of the skin, in much the same way that elastic fibers produce the rebound and good fit of a garment. If these fibers are denatured by chemical or mechanical means, such as ultraviolet exposure or stretching, a loss of elasticity results. The chemical change that denatures collagen and elastin is called oxidation, and results in loss of the vital properties of the fibers. Just as tights become baggy and ill-fitting as they lose their elasticity, so does skin as collagen and elastic fibers break down. Loose-fitting skin produces everything from saggy eyelids to jowls and a turkey gobbler neck. Clearly, it is to our advantage to maintain the integrity of the collagen and elastic fibers, for they hold it all together.

The superficial layer of the skin is called the epidermis. It is an exceedingly thin layer, but it's the only part you can see, so it had better look good. Unfortunately for us, the sins of the body are on very visible display here. The deepest portion of the epidermis is called the basal layer. It is virtually the only living portion of the epidermis. It produces a layer of cells, called keratinocytes, that migrate upward toward the surface, gradually being transformed into a protective coat of dead cells, called the keratinized layer, or stratum corneum, which in healthy, young skin is shed before it heaps up. In older skin the shedding process is slowed and a range of skin irregularities may result.

It is this most superficial component of the epidermis that acts as a barrier to the outside environment, and is always on display. It shows the wrinkles, gets sunburned, becomes scaly, blotchy, and dry, and when not properly cared for, makes our skin look weather-beaten and old. This keratinized layer is what we moisturize to the tune of hundreds of millions of dollars each year. But it is not money wasted, because the dead cells of the keratinized layer plump up when water is applied and sealed in with a layer of moisturizer. This effect lasts up to twelve hours, and actually makes the skin look smoother, and healthier. It is a fleeting and superficial treatment, but it has a place. Using moisturizers and makeup without treating the skin is much like covering a stale cake with fresh frosting.

In younger skin, the keratinized layer is shed regularly. The cells don't accumulate, and the epidermis functions as it was intended, as a protective barrier and mirror to the underlying dermis. One of the strategies we will employ is to effectively exfoliate the keratinized layer and keep it supple, youthful, and wrinkle-free. This is a simple route to smooth, blemish-free skin.

The epidermis and dermis together make up the skin. They are integrally related to one another and crucial to our existence. The skin, as a whole, acts as a barrier against loss of body water and dehydration, and as protection from the entry of bacteria into the body. It helps regulate body temperature by releasing perspiration, which evaporates and cools the skin, and by dilation of the blood vessels to release heat through direct transfer from the skin to the external environment. Constricting the blood flow in the skin retains heat when that is called for. In this respect, the skin is a functioning body organ, and it is critical to maintain its integrity. Even as the skin ages, it continues to perform these vital functions well.

The aging process is the sum of many factors. Chemical denaturing and oxidation of the collagen layer of the dermis is a naturally occurring phenomenon. It stretches, becomes less elastic, and sags. Constant usage also breaks down collagen in areas where it is folded, causing wrinkles. The blood supply to the skin, even without disease, becomes somewhat decreased and causes decreased nutrition and further breakdown of the collagen. Sun exposure accelerates collagen breakdown, and causes direct damage in the form of keratoses and skin cancer.

Various activities stretch the skin, including such benign things as leaning on one's palm while talking on the phone, or pulling at the skin with a towel. Soon enough the elastic fibers break down. With time the skin thins, loosens, discolors, and wrinkles. Not a pretty picture.

All the knowledge we have accumulated about aging cannot stop the process, but we *can* avoid accelerating it, and even slow it down. We can even control the signs and symptoms of aging before they start. And you can keep looking your best right through the very enjoyable middle years, but you must start early. The earlier the better. Unfortunately, the sad fact is that *wrinkles are forever*. The objective is prevention. Once wrinkles are written into the skin, they can never be fully eliminated. Though we can now reduce the depth of wrinkles and make them less apparent, they still remain a singular reminder of the wear and tear one suffers over the years. Therefore, we must prevent them before they start. That is truly the initial thrust of this program, and you will learn much more about the subject later. Nothing can completely eliminate a deep wrinkle once it has set. Facial folds and loosening, which are also manifestations of collagen and elastin breakdown, respond more favorably to surgery than wrinkles, but they too are better controlled prior to becoming full-blown.

Having performed thousands of face-lifts over these twenty years, I make it clear to my patients that it will be impossible to eliminate all their wrinkles. It is possible to make skin fit properly, rejuvenate it and eliminate blemishes, open the sagging eyes, reduce the deep skin folds and generally make them look as if they are only just beginning to age. And, of course, I always hope to produce a marked improvement. But I never cease to be saddened by those twenty years the patient spent helplessly watching the looseness and wrinkling become severe enough to require surgery. Those years were wasted waiting for the signs of facial aging to become more pronounced. Worse still, and frustrating for doctor and patient alike, some of those things can never be fully reversed. It becomes all the more apparent that the time to pay attention is now. This theme cannot be emphasized enough, and I will return to it repeatedly until it becomes as inevitable as aging itself. Our objective is maintaining your good looks. Follow the routine, make the little changes at the right time, and you may be lucky enough to keep looking great and never need a face-lift.

Back to the facts. Early aging shows first around the eyes. That is the thinnest skin of the face, and the most vulnerable to allergy, swelling, crying, and the wear and tear of expression. Next comes the deepening of the nasolabial fold. That is the line from outside the nostril to the corner of the mouth. Vertical frown lines between the eyebrows begin to show. Slight lines lead down from the corners of the mouth, sometimes accompanied by tiny pouches of fat. The occasional swelling beneath the eyes become bags and the smile lines deepen. An occasional vertical line develops in the upper lip. Horizontal forehead lines may develop, or deepen. Upper-eyelid skin becomes stretched and hooded, making you appear tired when you are not. Some wrinkles appear on cheeks, along with a few discolored spots. The lines leading down from the corners of your mouth seem to approach the jawline, giving the impression of jowls. The nasolabial lines deepen and a bit of fullness and loosening develops in the lower face and under the jaw. We could follow the process further, but you get the picture. The sum of these changes, if you allow them to develop, would require full face-lift and eyelid-lift to undo. Despite all that, the deep wrinkles would persist. Depending on one's genetic makeup, all this would typically take place by fifty-five to sixty years of age.

But why sit idly by and watch it coming, when a little self-help and a little maintenance can keep you in the Youth Corridor and looking great? True, you would have had to pay attention to lifestyle and skin care over the years, and yes, for the absolute optimal results you may actually need some form of cosmetic surgery along the way, but you will have looked your best for those important years from thirty-five to fifty-five, or sixty. You won't be wrinkled or sagging, and you can continue to look the way you feel: young, healthy, and attractive.

FIVE

PREVENTION

**very
important
dos and don'ts**

Understanding when to begin the routine is not very difficult. It's much like dressing for the day. The sensible person chooses clothing according to the weather, not the calendar. So should it be with seeking advice on a topic such as this. Don't wait for your thirty-fifth birthday, and don't wait until changes are obvious. The worst that could happen in seeking help too early is that you will be reassured and will have opened up a line of communication that will later prove invaluable. When I tell my patients they are not proper candidates for a particular surgical procedure, I emphasize the fact that my business is doing surgery, not denying it. If I think a procedure is inappropriate, they should recognize the honesty of the response. Human nature being what it is, often this advice is ignored, and patients go from doctor to doctor until they hear what they wish to hear. If you want surgery, you will certainly find someone willing to perform it, but it is not always the answer.

You have nothing to lose and everything to gain by making small lifestyle alterations and beginning early maintenance. So let us get started.

The first, and most important, step is taking a close and critical look at yourself. If you haven't already done that, then in all likelihood you are either too young to care, or your appearance is simply unimportant to you. There are probably people truly of the latter persuasion, but they are few and far between. Usually the disclaimer is a cover for an unfortunate sense of futility, behind which those least able to face facts will hide. To some significant degree most of us do care. Tastes and styles vary, and you may not be willing to commit yourself to this sort of endeavor, but I believe the majority of you have interest enough to read on. The ultimate objective is to prevent the changes of aging, not treat them. It all depends on where you enter the loop.

Back to that first look. If there are irregular areas of color or texture on your skin, and you need the help of moisturizers or cosmetics to return its lost luster, then the changes of adulthood have begun and it is the time to start. Fine lines about your eyes are early signs as well, but definitely time to get started. Up to this point, you can actually achieve great results with skin applications alone. If frown lines or smile lines are becoming part of your face, you're a bit past the self-help stage; nothing major is needed, but it is time to start. If there is a hint of the family double chin, it is time to deal with the problem while the easiest solutions and the best results are possible. All of these are among the early visible signs of aging, and respond well to the most basic care: in some cases, over-the-counter topical agents; in others, medical treatments; and in yet others, minor surgical procedures.

If you want to forestall further changes, this is the time to begin dealing with the issues. Perhaps no professional care need be added to your routine at this point, and very likely you can do much for yourself right here, with dramatic and long-lasting results. You're getting the drift. Start now.

Prevention is the first step. Ultimate regulation of the aging process is very likely genetic. Our intrinsic aging speed is determined by numerous hereditary factors, as well as our individual response to aging accelerators in the environment, particularly the number one culprit, sunlight. All together, these factors are responsible for the individual pace of aging. At some point, for everyone, the machinery simply wears out and the skin loses its resilience, elasticity, and luster, and the signs of aging become visible. That point becomes increasingly philosophical as science edges forward and aging is pushed farther along the curve. As far as the skin is concerned, there are both chemical and mechanical causes for the visible changes that we think of as aging, and we will be dealing with them in depth in the following pages.

The underlying mechanism of aging remains beyond our control in the preventative sense. We do know, however, that there is much in our behavior that can actually accelerate the aging process, and this should be avoided. The first step in maintenance is to delete negative forces from one's lifestyle. There are several specific dos and don'ts that are *imperative* to avoid making matters worse. Many of these you will already be aware of, some will surprise you, but all are important, all must be taken seriously if you wish to help yourself, and all are part of a simple, natural first step that should be part of your life before dealing with the strategies to follow. First the general rules.

1. DON'T SMOKE. Smoking constricts small blood vessels and reduces blood flow to the skin. The result is a decrease in nutrients and oxygen to the skin and an oxidation and denaturing of collagen. That causes loss of elasticity, sagging, and wrinkles. It's as simple as that. The evidence is so clear that most plastic surgeons won't perform face-lifts on smokers because the blood supply to the skin is so compromised that portions of the skin are actually at risk of dying. This problem doesn't appear in nonsmokers. That's how severe the damage can be. Add to that the vertical lines that develop in the lips from puffing away, and you can see some measure of the damage you are doing to yourself. All this without mentioning the risk of lung cancer and cardiovascular diseases so closely associated with cigarette smoking.

2. DON'T GAIN AND LOSE WEIGHT. Maintaining a relatively constant weight makes great sense for a volume of reasons. For our purposes, it is important to avoid the stretching of the skin caused by weight gain, and the laxity that follows weight loss. At some point, we can no longer get away with this. The skin loses just a touch of elasticity and doesn't snap back as quickly. That is the first warning signal. People in their thirties and forties are well advised to lose weight very slowly. Not simply for physiological reasons, but anatomically, in order to give the more slowly reacting skin a chance to shrink in size and fit the underlying structures closely and attractively. After a point, even this won't help. The skin will not respond to weight loss by shrinking, and will look loose, empty, and haggard. Not a very nice reward for having the fortitude to lose weight. The older you are, or the more weight you need to lose, the more likely this problem will arise. Weight loss of more than a few pounds should be at the rate of half a pound per week. It is quite acceptable to lose two or three pounds the first week, as that is primarily water. After that, moderation is crucial. The lesson, of course, is avoid significant weight gain, lose slowly, and above all, find your optimal weight and maintain it.

3. DON'T GET TOO THIN. Yes, you can be too thin. Hollow cheeks and thin skin may be fine for nineteen-year-old fashion models, but it makes an adult look frail and weak. There is nothing at all attractive about the cachectic look of anorexia. In fact, normal subcutaneous fat does much to plump out wrinkles and help the skin look and feel healthy. I am not proposing obesity, but you can surely be just too thin. Mental and physical health considerations aside, being excessively thin is simply unattractive in an overall sense.

4. DON'T RUN. I know everyone's doing it, but that doesn't make it right. At least don't be a long-term, long-distance jogger. Take a look at the serious runners you know who are in their mid-forties. Serious runners of normal weight have haggard, sunken faces due primarily to a loss of subcutaneous fat. It takes a while to manifest itself, but that is the price extracted for the benefits running offers.

Just as any weight loss, the total reduction of body fat that results from running affects the face first. First the face, then the breasts, then the buttocks and abdomen. Running is more specific still in the loss of facial padding. The constant rising and pounding down, rising and pounding down, lifts and pulls the facial skin away from the underlying muscles and bones. You surely have seen this in slow motion films of runners. The skin rises and falls and as the foot impacts, it continues to fall for another fraction of a second then bounces up again. The elastic fibers in the skin absorb the repeated trauma, until they eventually cease to fully bounce back, and ultimately stretch a bit, causing laxity of the skin. The combination of excessive loss of fat padding about the face and accelerated loss of elasticity have a decidedly negative impact on one's appearance. Jogging bras are universally worn for comfort and support against the tearing effect of the constant trauma of bouncing. The facial skin suffers the same fate, and goes unprotected. Add to that arthritic knees, ankles, and backs, and one would doubt running as the aerobic exercise of choice. It is not my intention to indict limited-frequency, limited-distance running, but be on guard. The beneficial effects of running are undeniable, but for most people biking or swimming or fast walking offers equal benefit and fewer pitfalls.

5. FACIAL EXERCISES ARE A WRINKLE WORK-OUT! DON'T DO THEM.

They cause wrinkles. The facial muscles, or muscles of facial expression, are that group of muscles that originate on the facial bones and end, or insert, at the skin. They are thin, flat muscles that are just beneath the skin and serve to animate the face, or give it expression; hence the name. To understand how they work, try this. Tighten the *orbicularis oculi* muscle. That's the muscle that encircles the eyes and makes up much of the bulk of the eyelids. Tightening the muscle makes you squint. Now do it again in front of the mirror. The squinting pulls the skin into wrinkles alongside your eyes. Now look in the mirror and smile and frown. The muscles of facial expression are attached to the skin, and repeated tightening, or exercising, of those muscles folds the skin over and over until wrinkles form.

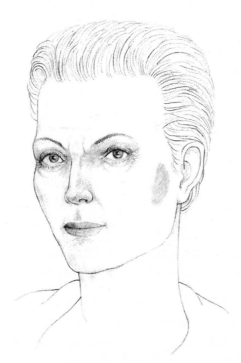

Notice smile lines at the corners of the eyes and on the cheeks and between eyebrows.
This is how facial muscles work.

Don't stop smiling. It's very human and very attractive, but that is a lot differ-ent than doing a wrinkle workout. The idea behind facial muscle exercises is surely well intentioned, but ignorant of anatomy. One day years ago, teaching the course in facial anatomy to a class of first-year medical students at Cornell Uni-versity Medical College, I whizzed through the anatomy of the muscles of facial expression, and prepared for questions. One of my students asked how the facial exercises, which had become quite popular, worked. It made me think, and I told them what I tell you. The muscular attachment to the skin is meant to graphi-cally reflect our expressions. Exercises in no way enhance the tone or strength of the skin, and when done repeatedly, indelibly etch wrinkles into the skin.

6. AVOID THE SUN. Nothing new or revolutionary here. Besides causing skin cancer, exposure to the sun is the primary accelerator of the break-down of collagen and elastic fiber, causing loosening and wrinkling of the skin. If all this wasn't enough, the sun also causes pigment changes, sunspots, and var-ious other unsightly eruptions. The intangible allure of a bit of color should be tempered with common sense, as there is absolutely no question that ultraviolet rays accelerate skin aging. Worse still, the effect is cumulative. Those days at the beach without sunblock will surely be paid for tomorrow, and the wise person would avoid adding today's insult to yesterday's injury.

7. NUTRITION. Change your diet! This absurd generalization is still far more universally applicable than it should be in our information-rich society. Since the majority of readers, women or men, are individuals concerned with their appearance, if not their health as well, one would expect this group above all others to understand and follow modestly healthy eating habits. Not true. The majority of Americans are overweight or on weight-gaining/losing seesaw diets. The naturally, metabolically thin individual can tolerate careless and unhealthy excessive-eating habits with impunity and not see the result for decades. The chronically overweight are bearing a potentially lethal load; and for different reasons, the chronically diet-thin present an equally precarious situation. That leaves a small number of well-nourished, consistently thin individuals, free of eating disorders and hormone imbalance.

The root of this ubiquitous problem lies with the basic American diet. Anyone old enough to be interested in this book has been nurtured on overindulging in an unhealthy pattern devised for us by authority figures and condoned by the government. A full measure of the burden of guilt lies with the medical profession at large: not intentionally of course, but by complicity and avoidance, compounded by lack of understanding and inadequate knowledge and attention to facts that one can hardly avoid. The leading cause of death among American males is heart disease. Women, especially postmenopausal women, are increasingly close behind. Among the root causes of the epidemic of heart disease is diet. Though the importance of other risk factors such as heredity, smoking, and lack of exercise cannot be denied, the fat-rich American diet is terminally related to the problem, and is a reversible component in many cases. Study after study shows the change in incidence of heart disease with introduction of Western, fat-rich diets. Asians, boasting a negligible incidence of heart disease, suddenly approach Western numbers as they assume Western dietary habits. Primitive cultures existing on high-vegetable, animal-fat-deprived diets are free of significant heart disease until they are introduced to the bounty of civilization. Examples are legion and the topic represents a book of its own. The point here is to direct you to reasonable eating habits. A diet that can kill you is certainly unhealthy. But it is unhealthy in so many insidious ways that the damage almost seems unrelated to the cause. We cannot easily register that the eating habits with which we grew up are wrong. We simply ingest too many calories for the work we do. We are continually overfueling the machine. And too much of the fuel is fat derived. Besides being a source of cholesterol and cholesterol building blocks, each gram of fat contains nine calories, while each gram of carbohydrate or protein contains only four. So in addition to basic health hazards, fat delivers more than twice the calories per unit of the other food sources. That alone is cause for change. We eat too much, and we eat too much of the wrong things.

The effect of all of this on one's appearance is both obvious and implied. Good health is of course reflected in one's appearance. Overweight and out of shape is not attractive. Assuming we all understand the value of proper weight mainte-nance, the appearance hazard is in cyclical gain and loss. Elastic and collagen fibers become increasingly unforgiving with the years. A twenty-pound weight fluctuation leaves loose skin in its wake. Small weight loss without rapid regain is well tolerated at any age. Larger weight loss must be spaced over months to allow the skin to compensate. Obviously, the greater the necessary loss, the less likely the skin will shrink to fit. The best tactic is to achieve one's optimal weight and stay there. That needn't be model slim or unrealistic for you, but a good and healthy level that your body can adjust to.

Over the years, I have given diet advice to innumerable patients. Several rules apply if one is to have any lasting success. The plan must be easy. There must be a sizable initial change to fire enthusiasm, and the goals must be clearly defined and within reach. The plans I might offer would likely be no more effective than those you have already tried, which speaks to the real problem. You shouldn't have needed more than one diet. Over the short haul they all work. Even four grapefruits and a prune a day will do the job for a week or two. The real issue is stabilizing your weight. That means forever. A fluctuation of three or four pounds is often seasonal or psychological, and perfectly acceptable. That is so because so small an amount, 2 percent of body weight, is easily shed without consequence. Maintenance requires a whole new mind-set. In order to be effec-tive it should require no thought at all once the changes have been learned. The following points have repeatedly proven their value. They are simple, painless, and in no way interfere with the enjoyment of food or the social aspects of meals.

1. **Begin your meal by drinking a full glass of water. It occupies volume and will slake some of the immediate hunger.**

2. **Eat salads as the first course instead of, according to the European tradition, after the main course. The purpose is obvious. Salad is filling and, bite for bite, lower in calories than anything that will follow.**

3. **Eat half of what is on your plate. You are no longer hungry, so why keep shoveling the calories in?**

4. **No second portions.**

5. **No desserts.**

6. **Between-meal snacks should be limited to low-calorie drinks, preferably water, and fresh fruit. An apple, in addition to tasting great, provides complex carbohydrates, which are digested slowly and, through feedback mechanisms, repress hunger far longer than prepared snacks made with refined sugar. Fresh fruit contains far fewer calories than snack food and is rich in vitamins, nutrients, and even naturally occurring antioxidants.**

Obviously, one should be concerned with the quality of food consumed. Fat and cholesterol in all forms should be controlled, and calories do count. Exercise, while burning calories during the act and even raising basal metabolic rate a bit for hours afterward, is not an excuse for overeating. An hour of tennis singles burns off barely 250 calories. Less than a Snickers and a Coke. Running a ten-minute mile consumes only 145 calories. Weight is controlled by ingesting only calories enough to support baseline body requirements plus physical work. This means far fewer calories than one would imagine. Happily, it can all be managed with ease if one is devoted to the task. Find a food chart and learn the basics. That will confirm what you already know about most foods. The rest is common sense. Find your own level and stick to it. The few tricks offered above will help, but remember, this is a maintenance aid, not a diet.

8. ANTIOXIDANTS AND FREE RADICALS. Two new scientific terms that have become unavoidable are *free radicals* and *antioxidants*. Free radicals are charged chemical particles of oxygen that enter into destructive chemical bonds with organic substances such as proteins. The result is an oxidation, or chemical burning, of the substance, which destroys it. Protein is denatured, genes may be broken, and dangerous residual substances may result from the chemical changes. All this has been going on for a very long time, though only recently has the process become a consuming interest of researchers and health faddists alike. At the same time that the destructive capabilities of free radicals were becoming known, many compounds that combat this destructive oxidation were identified. They are known as antioxidants, and include among their number many vitamins that were felt to be healthful even before the reasons were clarified.

Various activities of daily life have been shown to increase the presence of oxygen free radicals. These circulating, negatively charged particles have been associated with destructive oxidative activity. Exposure to sunlight is known to lead to oxidative destruction of the skin including increased incidence of skin cancer and processes causing wrinkling. Strenuous aerobic activity has been associated with free radical production leading to tissue damage. The evidence of oxidative damage caused by free radical production is real, and we are only just scratching the surface of understanding the mechanism. Along with the knowledge of the destructive capability of free radicals is the knowledge that they are products of normal metabolism, and are normally neutralized by antioxidant enzymes and diet-derived antioxidants. Included in this group are vitamin E, vitamin C (ascorbic acid), carotenes, and others. Vitamin E is the major nonenzymatic antioxidant protecting skin from the adverse effects of aging and sun damage. We don't know how much vitamin E is optimal for this function, or how to most effectively deliver it to the skin, but there is no scientific evidence that rubbing vitamin E onto the skin does any good at all. The molecule, as produced, is too large to penetrate the skin. Having said that, and at the risk of fueling baseless faddist theories, I am compelled to add that scientists at various centers are seeking ways to deliver vitamin E directly to the skin. There is also evidence that vitamins C and E are enhanced in their antioxidant function when present together above certain threshold amounts. Current conservative advice is that a diet rich in fruit and vegetables should be adequate for normal healthy adults. However, there is no evidence at all that 400 to 800 IU of daily additional vitamin E does any harm at all. In the past I believed vitamin E supplements unnecessary and perhaps worthless. The weight of new evidence has forced me to reconsider my position. It doesn't hurt, it very likely helps, and I encourage it. What seems necessary now is to determine the proper dosage and route of administration for maximal benefit.

Vitamin C has been given credit for all sorts of unproven miracles, and even some that have been proven. It is a potent antioxidant and a necessary component in tissue collagen production. Again, nutritionists and physicians advised that normal diets, including citrus fruit, provide adequate vitamin C. But there is evidence to the contrary. A series of well-known studies designed to prove or disprove the efficacy of vitamin C against the common cold showed it to reduce both the length of illness and the severity of symptoms. Interestingly, this was after a prior study denied efficacy. The second study utilized higher dosage and had positive results. This seems to show the dose-related nature of vitamin C, and has driven many people to live with massive doses. While probably not necessary, this is not harmful since excess vitamin C is quickly and harmlessly excreted in the urine. Most proponents believe that 1,000 milligrams per day is adequate for the desired antioxidant effect.

However, the matter has been further confused by a 1996 study, government supported through the National Institutes of Health, that has concluded that daily doses of vitamin C above 400 milligrams have no evident value. This conclusion is based on the body's ability to absorb vitamin C and the measured saturation of the white blood cells and plasma. The study also concludes that doses above 1,000 milligrams daily may promote the formation of kidney stones in some people.

Considering all these matters, I continue to recommend daily supplements of vitamin C of up to 1,000 milligrams.

The importance of vitamin C is well-known for its role in the healing of wounds and maintenance of the integrity of tissues. It is important in collagen synthesis, and its absence causes the disease scurvy, which results in tissue breakdown and open wounds. This was in the past a common condition suffered by sailors during long sea voyages. The association of citrus fruit with prevention of the disease led to British ships carrying stores of limes for consumption on extended passages, and hence the term *limey*.

With a solid background of scientific evidence and in the face of new miraculous claims for the effect of vitamin C on the skin, it is not surprising that it is showing up as an ingredient of many skin care preparations. The idea is to neutralize free radicals from the environment. Whether that takes place in significant amounts is questionable. Even more basic is the fact that environmental free radicals settling on the skin surface are probably not important at all. The ones outside can't get in. That is how the skin works. Real concern centers about the oxidative production of free radicals within the collagen of the skin, and the fact that vitamins C and E help reverse the damage. Stay tuned, there is more to come.

Beta carotene is another potent antioxidant for which numerous claims have been made. Among them, it has been suggested as active in the prevention of cholesterol oxidation, the process by which circulating cholesterol is changed to a form that sticks to the inside of arteries and blocks blood flow. In January of 1996 the results of two well-constructed, large studies found absolutely no benefit from beta carotene in prevention of heart disease. The studies also found an elevated death rate among smokers taking beta carotene. Whether this was serendipity or not, the use of this popular supplement has been discouraged.

If there is any antioxidant value of beta carotene to the skin it still has not been proven. However, both beta carotene and tretinoin (Retin-A) are closely related to vitamin A. The value of tretinoin in skin therapy seems assured, and beta carotene is a closely related compound, so is there something about all this that we don't yet understand? Very possibly. There is certainly food for thought, but for now, abandon beta carotene.

9. HORMONES. Hormones are integrally involved with the overall state of bodily affairs. Diseases excluded, there are changes in certain hormone levels that are predictably associated with aging. Just as testosterone levels decrease in the aging male, so estrogen levels in females dip slowly through adult life, finally reaching symptomatic levels at menopause. The importance of estrogen is well-known beyond hot flashes and loss of childbearing ability. Heart disease incidence of postmenopausal women nearly equals that of men of the same age, in contradistinction to the very low premenopausal incidence. Apparently, estrogen has a profoundly protective effect against heart disease. Estrogen withdrawal is followed rapidly by skin changes as well. Dryness, marked wrinkling, and loss of skin quality are the hallmarks. These are but two of the changes, but they are striking and important to consider. Both are preventable, and perhaps reversible with estrogen therapy. Unfortunately, that is only half of a complicated and incomplete story.

Estrogen replacement therapy dramatically reduces cardiovascular risk. It does, however, increase the risk of uterine cancer, among other potential problems. In women who have undergone hysterectomy and therefore have no uterus, the risk of uterine cancer is absent and estrogen replacement therapy is usually suggested for its cardiovascular protective effects and skin-salvaging qualities. The overwhelming preponderance of women undergo natural menopause and therefore suffer increased risk of uterine cancer with estrogen therapy alone. For cardiovascular protection this presents a dilemma. Should one undergo estrogen therapy and protect the heart and skin at the expense of increased uterine risk? Most evidence points to combining estrogen with progestin for the most natural replacement. A recent federally funded study found that this combination provides cardiovascular protection and very significantly reduces uterine risk, helping to clarify the direction of therapy. Unfortunately, estrogen replacement may also be associated with increased risk of breast cancer. It remains unclear whether combined therapy will neutralize that risk as well. The debate rages on.

The newest estrogen-related information comes from a large-scale, long-term Harvard study published in August 1996. The results of this study infer that estrogen is significantly important in preventing Alzheimer's disease. A marked reduction in the incidence of the disease was noted among postmenopausal women on estrogen replacement therapy compared to the untreated group. This appears to be good news indeed.

Estrogen replacement therapy will keep your skin looking better, but there is more to the choice than that. The decision for estrogen replacement should not be taken lightly. There exists a wealth of conflicting and confusing information, and more surfaces daily. Currently, estrogen and progestin replacement therapy is the route of choice for most women. If this issue applies to you, the best source of information should be your gynecologist. It is an issue they deal with on a daily basis with patients and professional colleagues. Though most gynecologists are up-to-date on the newest studies, opinions still vary. You and your doctor will have to weigh the information, and ultimately you must decide for yourself.

[THINK ABOUT IT]

After you have had time to digest the importance of these general rules, you will be able to benefit greatly by incorporating them into your own life situations. If you are reading this book with your elbow on your desk, your cheek cradled in your hand, you are passively stretching the skin of your cheek. The same applies to telephone time. It may not seem like a big deal, but it adds up to repeated inadvertent fatiguing of the elastic fibers, and it definitely takes its toll. Ultimately, loss of skin elasticity is accelerated. It doesn't happen overnight, but it happens.

If you are saying, "I don't sit with my cheek in my hand," you are not paying attention. Think of similar situations that might apply to you. Do you habitually pull at the skin of your neck? Lots of people do, and you can guess where it leads. Do your eyelids swell when you drink red wine or eat spicy foods? Enough stretching and swelling will result in damage to the delicate skin of the lids, and permanent stretching and looseness will result. How much of this will cause damage? That is impossible to quantify. It would be difficult to find human volunteers wishing to have their skin stretched out of shape. Suffice it to say, the process of aging and loss of elasticity will be accelerated. Think about it, and use common sense in your lifestyle decisions. Changing these unimportant habits is not terribly painful. One spicy pizza, a few pulls on the skin, and occasional cheek cradling are not going to change your life, but make a point of thinking about what you do. Change your habits; reduce the insults to your skin. Nothing here requires the soul of a zealot nor the self-denial of a Buddhist monk. Simply make an effort not to make things worse.

what's OUT THERE

**a survey of
lotions, potions,
and treatments—
some good,
some bad**

In the best of all possible worlds, the ultimate goal of this effort would be to teach people how to stay young. That is not reality, for only a tiny portion of the population is young enough to learn to control aging before the signs appear. For the great majority, that means helping those with visible signs of aging to reset the clock and start again. Toward this end, you will soon learn effective strategies for dealing with a wide range of problems, many of which require no medical care. We have touched upon the basic dos and don'ts, so that everyday life may work for us, not against us. Now we must consider actually making an effort to help ourselves. The easiest and most logical place to launch is into the world of skin care and treatment. Originally, skin care and treatment were two distinct worlds. So much overlap currently exists that separation is no longer productive. This section covers effective skin care products that are available over-the-counter without doctor's prescription. Whenever possible, I will omit trade names and stick to functional grouping and active ingredients. In a few cases, this will be impossible.

The advertising pages of fashion magazines and the skin care section of stores provide a virtual assault of promises and claims. Strangely enough, some of them are true. That was not always the case, and today's skin care world is a far cry from the old "promise in a pot." Unfortunately, you mustn't let down your guard, for numerous useless additives and false promises still abound. But things have changed, and for the better. Among the big changes have been the addition of alpha hydroxy acid and sunblock to many over-the-counter lines. Until recently, there was little that over-the-counter preparations could actually change. Moisturizers worked well as long as one expected a simple twelve-hour hydration of the keratinized layer of the skin. In that case, it was a promise kept. That was the level of therapy one could expect. All the claims for special penetrating moisturizing droplets and skin-rejuvenating enzymes were absolute nonsense. None of the preparations actually penetrated the dermis, or in any way changed the nature of the skin. If they did so to any significant extent, they would be considered drugs by the FDA, and require a doctor's prescription. But the use of alpha hydroxy acids, along with sunscreens and moisturizers, has provided the basis for intelligent programs that actually make a difference. In a sense, these products are revolutionary. They work. Still, they are not a magic bullet, and require intelligent and dedicated usage to be effective. Read through the chapter. All the information will be incorporated in specific examples and maintenance routines later in the book.

[Alpha Hydroxy Acids]

Alpha hydroxy acid (AHA) preparations are available over-the-counter, without prescription. Currently, the Food and Drug Administration has no restrictions on the concentration of AHA in over-the-counter or skin care salon preparations. The only applicable rule is that the product not cause harm. Most products offer concentrations of up to 10 percent AHA, which are useful and safe. Alpha hydroxy acids in higher concentration can cause actual peels with all the attendant side effects. Therefore, the manufacturers are wisely avoiding the risk of a more potent concentration. Conversations between my staff and the FDA lead us to believe that some sort of regulation is not far off, and that is good. Meanwhile, over-the-counter product manufacturers are encouraged to maintain a concentration below 10 percent AHA. That concentration is quite safe, and although it does not provide actual therapeutic peeling, the constant desquamation, or shedding of surface cells, that does take place, smooths the skin. It softens superficial wrinkles and partially reverses sun damage. Medical AHA peels use a concentration of 30 to 70 percent, the effects are more dramatic, and they must be dealt with more carefully. We will refer to this type of AHA peel as therapeutic or concentrated, to avoid confusion with the over-the-counter products being discussed in this section. Most over-the-counter product manufacturers use concentrations of 7 or 8 percent. Some of the AHA groups seem effective in even lower concentrations. The resulting decrease in efficacy is balanced by the reduced risk of actual peeling or irritation from the acid. That makes it an excellent maintenance tool for those who have undergone more concentrated medical-level peels and want to perpetuate the effect, and is a fine daily refresher for those who do not yet need a true peel.

Alpha hydroxy acids are derived from naturally occurring substances, such as sugarcane, citrus fruit, grapes, and milk, and are known as glycolic acid, lactic acid, citric acid, salicylic acid, or others, depending on the source. The active ingredient is an alpha hydroxy acid, hence the generic term. As far as I can determine from personal observation and the scientific literature, there is little difference which acid type is used, as long as it is produced properly, of the proper concentration, and applied properly.

Alpha hydroxy acids come in many forms. Manufacturers have mixed them with moisturizers, sunblocks, and who knows whatever else. This serves to complicate and confuse a simple plan. You should stick to the purest products. Use alpha hydroxy acids as they were intended, as exfoliants. The acid can be delivered in many forms. The choice of cream, gel, lotion, or dilute wash is said to be based on the oil level of the skin. Here too, too many choices confuse the issue. To point yourself in the right direction, consider this. The maintenance product provided by your dermatologist or plastic surgeon for maintainence after concentrated alpha hydroxy acid peels is of about the same strength as the cosmetic company model and is not altered for skin type. Sure, there might be the individual whose skin becomes excessively dry from an AHA lotion, but these variations are slight and rare. We find that either the product is tolerated or it is not. The presenting vehicle, and the cosmetic counter analysis to choose the right one, is an unnecessary conceit.

Essentials of the alpha hydroxy acid story are these. Low-concentration AHA products are effective in improving the appearance of the skin. Various formulations containing from 2 to 8 percent AHA are available. They speed the shedding of the superficial keratinized layer of the skin, resulting in a more regular skin surface; lighten blemishes; and improve very superficial wrinkles and sun damage. At this strength it will not tighten the skin or eliminate wrinkles, but long-term use offers significant improvement in the overall look of the skin.

The first reported devotee of alpha hydroxy acid was probably Cleopatra, who covered her face with wine as a beauty treatment. Grapes, and therefore wine, are a source of AHA. If it worked for Cleopatra, what took us so long to catch up?

Don't confuse the use of this low-concentration AHA with therapeutic AHA peels. They are decidedly different in their intent and result. The regular use of

AHA at home over a period of months will improve the look of your skin. The medical application of a series of 50 to 70 percent AHA peels will eliminate many superficial wrinkles, smooth the skin, truly reverse visible sun damage and discoloration, and may actually improve the underlying collagen and elastic tissues. These are related treatments for decidedly different circumstances, and will be covered in depth in the section on peels. Here we are concerned with effective home treatment in a skin care routine.

The products are best used from several times a week, to daily, over a period of at least several months. The frequency of use should increase with age and need. Continual daily usage has been very well tolerated among my patients, though I believe a rest period each year is useful. The least concentrated preparations are most suitable for daily usage. Extended application is important, but so is the rest period. Because application every day, or every evening, seems to work, that doesn't mean that twice-daily application is better. The AHAs are irritants, and work by dislodging the superficial layer of the skin and encouraging a more rapid cell turnover. A frequent complaint is excessive redness and irritation. If you are lucky enough to avoid this problem with normal usage, don't look for trouble. The skin needs time for repair. Even if your skin responds perfectly, alternating periods of use and rest is advisable. Typically, the younger person should use AHA preparations every other night for six months followed by a month without treatment or three weeks out of every four, all year through. Frequency, and sometimes strength, are increased for older people and those with more damaged skin, who need the treatment more. At some point on the aging scale, the dilute acids aren't enough and a series of more concentrated AHA peels must be performed by the dermatologist or plastic surgeon. These are followed again by the long-term use of the milder solutions. Here we are discussing only the commercial preparations. The attitude one should take regarding use of alpha hydroxy acid is that as modest as the result may be, this is the first over-the-counter product that actually works.

The use of dilute AHA solutions should not be reserved solely for visible signs of aging. Periodic use for teenage and young adult skin helps remove debris and alleviate blackheads and whiteheads, and smooth irregular areas. Women in their twenties and thirties will see a smoothing, clearing effect, and if the theory of improved turnover of the keratinized layer of the epidermis is correct, they may see long-term benefits from early treatment.

Is it possible that early treatment may prevent or forestall aging of the facial skin? Perhaps. What we do know is that the skin surface improves, blemishes fade, and the collagen layer of the skin seems to improve. We haven't been at this long enough to say much else. Can there be negative effects from long-term AHA use? Anything is possible, but so far there have been no significant reports of risk. Studies continue and the FDA surely keeps an eye opened, but so far all reports are positive. Regular use of alpha hydroxy acids appears beneficial for young and old alike. It will be fascinating to watch the long-term effect of this treatment on people who start at age twenty-five and continue usage for decades. Will their skin defy normal aging? How much better will they fare than their peers who did nothing until the signs of aging were undeniable? Stay tuned. Meanwhile, twenty-five or fifty-two, this should become part of your routine.

[SUNSCREENS]

Aside from disease states and the intrinsic, genetically determined changes that fall within the category of skin aging, experts regularly identify and implicate only two external causes for the phenomenon. They are sun exposure and cigarette smoking. It's as simple as that. No hedging, no modifying, no softening the blow.

In 1988 the American Academy of Dermatology stated that the majority of undesirable clinical features associated with skin aging are the result of damage due to ultraviolet radiation. That is basically sunlight and excludes X rays and other forms of radiation. Ultraviolet light is divided into groups based on the wavelength of the light. We are concerned primarily with the bands of light called ultraviolet A and ultraviolet B (UVA and UVB). They are closely related and the spectrum of one melds into the spectrum of the other. UVA is much more prevalent in the environment, but a thousand times less effective at causing skin injury. There is more UVA radiation in the atmosphere, but UVB is more destructive, and responsible for the majority of sunburn, skin cancer, and skin aging. Therefore, we must protect against both. UVB radiation is largely absorbed by the ozone layer of the atmosphere. We know the ozone layer is becoming depleted due to chronic pollution, and the incidence of skin cancer is proportionally on the rise. The accelerated skin aging from UVB exposure is not as easily measured as the numbers of skin cancers per year, but since the same insult stimulates both processes, it too must be on the rise.

Exposure to the sun causes a whole range of reactions. Some are immediately detectable and predictable. There is an immediate reddening phase followed by burning in some people and tanning in others. Gradual exposure to the sun affords protection from burning in many individuals, particularly those with darker skin. This ability to tan varies from person to person, but can be traced ultimately to one's genetic origins. As a rule, fair-skinned northern Europeans suffer sunburn while those of southern ancestry tend to tan. The dense pigment of African descent provides the most effective protection. All this is, of course, a rough generalization. We are no longer pure-bred anything and we must learn what is our own reaction to the sun by trial and error. Those with greater tanning ability are more tolerant of the sun, and the tan itself offers some measure of protection from some of the harmful effects of ultraviolet radiation. Nonetheless, sun-damaged skin, whether through tanning or burning, shows characteristic changes under the microscope. They are primarily degenerative changes within the collagen layer that result in loss of elasticity and wrinkling. The outer, epidermal, layer becomes hyperactive, thickening and causing irregularities and blotchy discoloration on the skin. All together, this coarse, loose, leathery, blotchy, wrinkled skin is called prematurely aged. The changes under the microscope are specific and can be clearly distinguished from the normal skin of an older individual. This is something we are doing to ourselves. It is unnecessary and it is avoidable.

In addition to the above, the most critical change is the very increased susceptibility to skin cancer. I have chosen the word *susceptibility* intentionally. There is no doubting the relationship of sun to skin cancer, but there is now some evidence that chronic sun exposure depresses the immune system and weakens the defenses against skin cancer. Though skin cancer and aging are not the same thing, both are so closely related to sun exposure that one should not think of one without the other.

The American Cancer Society estimates that more than 1 million new skin cancers will be diagnosed in the year 1996. Some 80 percent of these will be basal cell carcinomas, the most easily cured of all cancers, and usually not a significant health hazard. Most of these 800,000 cancers will have been caused by sun exposure. There are exceptions, but as a rule basal cell carcinomas are caused by the sun. A similar causal relationship exists for the next most frequent skin cancer, squamous cell carcinoma. The least numerous of these skin cancers is melanoma. Approximately 40,000 of these potentially lethal lesions will arise this year. Until not too long ago, there wasn't a causal relationship known between melanoma and sun exposure. Now it seems clear that not tanning but actual sunburn predisposes an area of skin to melanoma.

If all of this sounds frightening, it is meant to be. Think about this. Seventy-five percent of a person's ultraviolet exposure (sun) is accumulated before age twenty. And yet these skin cancers are a disease of middle age and older. Sun damage is a cumulative phenomenon. We pay for our sins long after the day at the beach. A study from the Harvard Medical School estimates that the use of effective sunscreen during the first eighteen years of life would reduce the level of nonmelanoma skin cancers by 78 percent. A very impressive number indeed. If you are fair skinned, then for no other reason than cancer protection, you must become a devoted user of sunscreen if you enjoy any outdoor activities at all.

Sun exposure is also the culprit in premature aging of the skin. It can not be said often enough. Having established a relationship beyond refuting we must decide how to manage the facts. There is no reason to deny yourself the enjoyment of the great outdoors. Nor is there reason to so restrict your lifestyle that the slightest tan becomes a source of concern. That is simply too extreme. However, you must protect yourself where you can. It does not make sense to sunbathe without adequate protection. You can learn to enjoy the regenerating feel of the sun without doing harm. It is not a terribly restricting concept. Wide-brimmed hats, sunscreens, and common sense are here to stay.

There are two categories of sunscreens. Physical sunscreens and chemical sunscreens. The former are like the white stuff the lifeguards put on their noses, zinc oxide, and do their job by acting as a physical barrier to the sun. These are effective at reflecting the light and thereby protecting the skin. They include titanium dioxide, iron oxide, magnesium silicate, and other opaque and reflective materials, which suffer from being difficult to prepare and difficult to apply in a pleasant and invisible coat.

Chemical sunscreens absorb the ultraviolet radiation as filters. Various chemicals protect against the spectrum of ultraviolet light. The most commonly used of these is para-aminobenzoic acid (PABA). Pure PABA use has become less popular due to the high incidence of allergy and irritation associated with it. Related compounds have taken up the slack. Frequently used active ingredients include oxybenzone, dioxybenzone, salicylates, cinnamates, and anthranilates. These are very effective, and if you pick up the sunscreen you currently use, you will find some of them listed among the ingredients. The package should also be clearly marked with the sun protection factor (SPF) of the product. The SPF refers to the laboratory-determined time required for skin to burn with sunscreen as opposed to the time required for the same level of sunburn without protection. A sunscreen that offers an SPF of 2 would allow an individual who would burn in 30 minutes to be exposed to the sun for 60 minutes before reaching the same level of sunburn. Likewise, the most popular SPF 15 products should allow the same individual 15 times 30, or 450, minutes of safe exposure. Does one application of SPF 15 really afford you more than seven hours of protection? Theoretically. In actual practice, however, it depends on how quickly you would burn without sunscreen, the conditions at the moment, how well and how thickly the sunscreen was applied, and whether it had been rubbed, washed, or sweated off. The SPF is only a guide. There are products available with ratings of 30 or higher, but laboratory values and actual practice are rarely the same. Some sunscreens are specifically formulated for people who tend toward clogged pores and acne, and others are more acceptable to children, who dislike the slight stinging associated with alcohol present in some lotions.

When picking a sunscreen you should check for these things:.

1. **SPF.**
2. **Active ingredients. Through trial and error you will eliminate products and ingredients that are unpleasant or irritating.**
3. **Water-resistant or waterproof. This is an important consideration for swimming or sports. Water-resistant means that the product continues to protect after forty minutes of immersion; waterproof, for up to eighty minutes. In the past these had been thicker or more difficult to spread than other products, but more recently they seem to have become more elegant. If you plan to spend time at the beach, they are certainly worth a try.**

Many manufacturers now offer combination sunscreen and moisturizer products. This is a useful idea if only because it simplifies routines and helps make using sunscreen a habit. Two questions arise. Do these formulations work as well and feel as good as moisturizer alone? Only you can make that determination regarding the aesthetic appeal of the product. And: Does one always need sunscreen twice daily, or as often as moisturizer? Probably not, but surprisingly, the best time to apply sunscreen is hours before it is necessary, so that it has time to interact with the keratinized top layer of the skin. It might be a good idea to apply a moisturizer/sunscreen at night. A lot depends on your lifestyle and where you live. Sunny climates and high altitudes require more protection on a daily basis than the bleak north at sea level. Assuming the combination moisturizer/ sunscreen is as effective as sunscreen alone, does the combination simplify or complicate developing a routine? It has always seemed to me that the combination products are good only if they simplify the daily baseline. Make them as much a part of the morning routine as brushing your teeth and alter and add to the routine as your activities demand.

[MOISTURIZERS]

Anything that can force the superficial keratinized layer of the skin to temporarily retain water is a moisturizer. These cells are no longer functioning, and are in the process of drying and flaking away. If they are not rubbed away or moisturized, they leave the skin with a dry, irregular, and superficially wrinkled surface. Applying water and sealing it in with a moisturizer hydrates and enlarges these cells, thus obliterating the wrinkled, irregular surface and making the skin appear temporarily healthier. There is nothing the least bit healthier about moisturized skin, but it does look better. That is quite a lot for what little goes into the process.

Commercially available moisturizers are either petroleum based or water based. They both work, though the oil-based products are often more effective and less elegant to the touch. Simple, familiar examples include Vaseline, but even Crisco will do. Though few would choose to apply the latter to their face, it would certainly do the job. Most choose among the well-formulated creams so readily available at cosmetic counters. Here the confusion begins. Collagen? No collagen? Special secret ingredient X? Or not? That is all beside the point and useless as far as moisturizing is concerned. Collagen in a cream does not get into your skin. Period. If you like the product, use it. But not because it contains collagen. The same is true for special ingredients of any sort: the exception being combination moisturizer/sunscreens, which are what they say they are. As far as moisturizers are concerned, find one that feels good, and use it.

Moisturizers are designed for twice-daily use. They are applied to moist skin and gently rubbed in. There should be no residue, and makeup can be applied directly to the skin. In some climates and situations, more frequent usage is necessary.

[GROWTH HORMONE]

This subject enters the realm of science fiction. Unfortunately, it seems that although the facts are pure science, the therapeutic results, alas, may be fiction, or at least wishful thinking. Since the seeds of probability do exist, small cults of believers have arisen. The use of growth hormone for rejuvenation has burst the confines of scientific conjecture, and landed on the front page of *The Wall Street Journal.* Claims of miraculous rejuvenation of every sort have been made. People are using it, people are making large sums of money providing it, and we should start at the beginning and try to understand the facts.

Human growth hormone is produced by the acidophilic cells of the anterior portion of the pituitary gland within the brain. This *master gland,* as it is called, functions by producing and circulating hormones that stimulate endocrine glands to produce hormones that affect bodily functions. Its signals set the adrenal and thyroid glands to work, and generally act to regulate hormone activity. One of the substances produced is growth hormone, which triggers activity in the growth centers of the bones, and in secondary supporting structures, such as muscles. Not very long ago it was found that children and young adults with stunted growth could be pushed toward normal by the injection of growth hormone. The success of the therapy was dependent on the relatively low level of the hormone produced naturally. It was a big step forward, but was relegated to treatment of growth defects. It was also known that in normal individuals, growth hormone production drops off rapidly after adolescence; however, a continual level can be expected throughout adulthood. Some adults have lower levels than others of growth hormone, and from here sprung the seed for an interesting study. A small number of men in their fifties and sixties with reduced levels of circulating growth hormone were treated with injections of the substance, and their progress monitored. The results varied from interesting to surprising.

The subjects reported a general sense of well-being and mood elevation. Interesting, but not a big deal. Lots of substances of real and imagined potency can do that. But an increased bone density and a measurable increase in muscle mass also accompanied treatment. Instead of wasting with age, these men were growing, bulking up, showing increased sexual activity, and in short, responding in an age-defying manner from libido to skin texture. Exciting? You bet. But don't start getting injections yet. There is more to the story.

Unfortunately, the studies done to date were very small, and very inconclusive. Some of the negative side effects noted were breast development in males, carpal tunnel syndrome (a painful and debilitating entrapment of the median nerve at the wrist), and other minor and treatable symptoms. "So what," you say. "I'll gladly have those treated, and stay young forever."

Not so fast. Another reported side effect from the growth hormone treatment is grotesque overgrowth of the face. The bones actually enlarge and the features expand. That is not such good news. Prudent investigators put it all together and needed time for reevaluation. Charlatans and dreamers moved full steam ahead. I find the whole subject fascinating, and I am convinced that you will be hearing more and more about this exciting and dangerous dream in the very near future. My advice? Wait and see. Too many people have been stimulated by the possibilities for it to go unexplored, but don't take a risk that could be devastating. Keep your eyes open and your brain working; we will know much more about it soon enough.

SEVEN

a skin care routine

THAT WORKS

Here is what you will need:

1. **Soap and water**
2. **Moisturizer**
3. **Sunscreen**
4. **Alpha hydroxy acid preparation**
5. **Cleanser**
6. **Tretinoin (Retin-A)**

A good skin care routine must make sense, and it must work. A proper routine should function on several levels. Superficially, pure cleansing is critical. That means the ability to remove the daily grit buildup of the modern environment, as well as the constantly produced crop of cellular debris and surface oils. Those oils are both fresh and denatured, and cannot be readily separated from one another. Optimally, one should remove the oxidized oils and preserve the fresh skin oil, with its natural moisturizing qualities. That cannot be effectively done, and at some point it is advisable to remove the combination of existing oils and start fresh. Once the oil and debris are cleansed away, the routine must provide for remoisturization. That is again a superficial solution, but it looks good and it feels good. Next, trouble areas must be addressed. Fine wrinkles, color changes and blotches, and surface irregularities tilt the equation. Then, on the deepest level, the routine must do whatever possible to maintain and improve the infrastructure of the skin. All these functions must be combined in a soothing, easily learned, and rewarding process. No matter how good the routine, if you don't follow it, it is useless.

There are many variables to consider, but some aspects apply to all. Cleansing, exfoliating, moisturizing, and sun protection are a must. Other possibilities are discussed on an individual basis. At the end of this section, you will see the step-by-step directions for your twice-daily home skin care. This routine alone will make your skin more youthful and attractive. It is the launching pad for the rest of the options. If you do nothing more than these simple steps, you will have made great and visible strides. Healthy skin looks and reacts better. It will hold up longer and even respond to procedures with better results than uncared-for skin.

Start by washing with soap and water. This is not heresy; it is common sense and good advice. Rich soap lather is the best vehicle for removing old oils, cellular debris, and environmental residue, including cosmetics. Much of this is the source of irritation and irregularity of the skin. If you are going to take a skin care routine seriously, you might as well know what is present on your skin, what has been washed away, and what needs to be added. Certainly there are people whose skin is so dry and delicate that washing with soap and water is an aggravating exercise. Fortunately, these people are few and far between. Most have mixed areas of oily, dry, and normal skin, with the nose and forehead and eyebrow area being the oiliest, the cheeks the driest. To complicate matters further, these diverse areas vary in their moisture qualities according to climate and activities. Anxiety, stress, hard work, and especially sex have a profound effect on oil production and the relative moisture of the skin. As a rule, the skin becomes drier as we age, and accommodation should be made for this on an individual basis. Generally, we cannot predict the state of hydration of the skin from month to month, or from hour to hour. It helps our planning to know what we are actually dealing with. To do that, we must return to *ground zero*. Clean all external substances from the skin surface, treat as necessary, moisten, and seal in the moisture with a moisturizer.

Rinse your face with water that feels warm to the touch. It should not actually be hot. Remember that body temperature is 98.6 degrees Fahrenheit. Therefore, any water temperature above 98.6 degrees will feel warm. That's all you need. The water must be warm enough to encourage vasodilation and encourage blood supply. It must also be warm enough to soften skin oils and debris. That will help the lather clean residual makeup, oxidized skin oils, and ambient pollution and cellular debris from the skin surface.

Lather generously with a mild soap of slightly acidic pH. The surface of the skin should be slightly acidic and it makes little sense to upset it. Basis and Dove, among other soaps, are excellent as far as balance and gentleness are concerned. Avoid soaps with perfume. Some seemingly mild soaps are too basic for the skin, and leave residue. Others contain antibacterial formulations, which may be an irritant to certain skin types, as well as perfumes, which are definitely of no therapeutic value. The rule of thumb is to choose a brand that feels good, lathers well in your local water, and seems to wash off without leaving residue. Even if you make a mistake and choose the least effective soap, your skin will still be cleaner and freer of debris than had you used cleansing creams or lotions alone.

Gently rub the lather over the skin of the face and neck. Don't forget the eyelids. This should take only thirty seconds.

Wash the lather off with copious amounts of warm water.

Repeat the process. This time follow the warm water rinse with a refreshing final rinse with cold water. That will close down the blood vessels, firm the skin, and it feels great. When moisturizer alone is used, it should be applied to still-moist skin. Alpha hydroxy acid or Retin-A (tretinoin), when indicated, is applied to totally dry skin. A twenty-minute waiting period is advised between washing and Retin-A use. Moisturizer is applied after Retin-A.

A note about skin cleansers. There is a place for these nonsoap cleansers. Those specifically designed to remove makeup, particularly mascara, are quite useful. They will do very well at this task, but do not consider them a substitute for soap and water. We approach our skin care routine from *ground zero*. That means getting all surface contamination off. Washing with soap and water does this best. If you are worried about soap being too dry and can't wait a minute and a half for the application of moisturizer, then use one of the newer, superfatted facial soaps.

This is a good place to talk about how much cream and lotion is enough. Moisturizers, sunscreens, and treatments should be applied to the skin surface and gently rubbed in. All evidence of the cream should disappear. There should be no surface residue, no slippery greased feeling. There is no advantage to be gained from using more than the thin layer that disappears readily into the surface of the skin. You should not see it, and it should not feel greasy.

Use your towel for exfoliation. After showering or washing your face, towel briskly. This should be done at least once a day. The process helps remove heaped-up dead skin cells and allows the healthy young cells to reach the surface. Toweling should always be done in the down-to-up direction to avoid stretching the skin downward with gravity. Be gentle with yourself. The towel will do a great job with virtually no pressure at all. It feels good and your skin will assume a healthy glow. This results from the irritation of even the gentlest rubbing of the skin surface. The glow retreats rapidly and no harm is done by this gentle exfoliation.

Moisturizer. After the morning wash, and before applying makeup or moisturizer, sunscreen should be applied. This is a routine that works best when it doesn't vary. Surely you will not suffer significant ultraviolet damage to your skin in a Chicago February, commuting by car to an indoor workspace. You are safe to eliminate this step. But when do you begin again? The only routines that work are ones that become routine. When you find a sunscreen that is easily tolerated, use it every day. Makeup or moisturizers containing sunscreen are excellent for this purpose.

Moisturize after the sunscreen and onto moistened skin. The need for moisturizer often varies inversely with the need for sunscreen. When the weather is cold and you retreat to the heated indoors, you have little need for sunscreen. The same circumstances are powerful drying influences. Cold air with very low humidity and superheated, dry indoor air desiccate skin, and increase the need for moisture treatment.

Moisturizers and the process of moisturization of the skin is a fleeting proposition indeed. The actual moisture content of the skin as a whole varies little under normal circumstances. The function of moisturizing compounds is to trap moisture in the superficial skin layer of dead keratinized cells. The nature of this layer varies from dry and scaly, to smooth and healthy appearing, depending on the amount of moisture temporarily trapped within. The whole thing is somewhat artificial. On the other hand, the process is mimicking the end point of the natural process. Individuals producing greater amounts of skin oils are in effect sealing the moisture into the keratinized layer with the body's own moisturizer. This substance lasts longer than most moisturizers, and actually must be washed away periodically. Equally potent moisturizers could be easily produced but they would be poorly tolerated and inelegant, to say the very least. As we mentioned previously, Crisco would be very effective, but not on the top of anyone's list.

For these reasons, we use pleasant, well-tolerated moisture creams, and replenish them twice a day. It is incorrect to think of these ubiquitous creams as treatment, for they do not penetrate the skin or effect any permanent change on the skin surface. Nonetheless, they play an important role in the overall plan. Though they offer no actual therapeutic value, one cannot deny that they make the skin look and feel better. That won't keep you young forever, but it will help you look your best each day.

Alpha hydroxy acid or tretinoin cream (Retin-A). This should be applied, after washing and toweling dry, and should be followed by the application of moisturizer. As mentioned above, it is important to apply tretinoin to thoroughly dry skin, and a waiting period after washing is advised. These are once-a-day applications and are most easily performed at night. The exception is when both are being used simultaneously. In that case, one usually applies the AHA preparation in the morning, and tretinoin at night. The alpha hydroxy acid preparation may be contained in a moisturizer vehicle, and will save a step without sacrificing efficacy. Tretinoin cream, the active ingredient in Retin-A and Renova, is available only by prescription, and is discussed under medical treatments.

This basic routine is simple enough, and probably varies very little from your current routine. The use of active ingredients such as tretinoin and alpha hydroxy acids is the big step forward. The routine alone will not stop the clock, but it will make a definite and cumulative difference.

trouble spots and

TREATMENT

Now that we have established the dos and don'ts, and a proper skin care routine to follow, it is time to help you wherever you cannot help yourself. This is a most innovative place, for here we will identify the trouble spots, hopefully before they arrive, and deal with them before they cause indelible changes. This is newer thinking. It is aimed at minimal intervention and maintenance. If you begin early and follow this schedule through the years, you may never need more than minor procedures to keep looking your best. If you begin at forty or later, it may ultimately lead to a face-lift, which you may accept or reject, but you will surely look far better along the way than had you not followed the program. In fact, that applies to any stage. You will always benefit from the effort and interest you have spent. Despite the fact that aging ultimately rears its unwelcome head, you will *always* look better than your identical twin who didn't follow the program. Some of the techniques we will explore are relatively new; most have been around for a while. All have been primarily thought of as ancillary procedures; often they have been thought of only when surgery is considered later in life. In my practice I have found it useful to isolate these procedures and apply them individually as trouble spots surface. I find that these small procedures are far more useful for keeping younger people young. Save your face-lift for your sixtieth birthday.

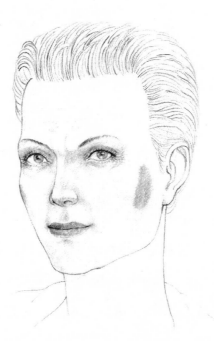

This drawing illustrates many changes listed here.

The following is a list of annoying changes that will manifest themselves at different times for different individuals. Don't worry, you won't have them all, and they won't all happen at once. I have tried to follow the chronological order of appearance, keeping the worst for last. Don't sneak a look at the mirror and get depressed.

1. **Smile lines outside eyes**
2. **Fine wrinkles under eyes**
3. **Fine wrinkles on cheeks**
4. **Dry or blotchy skin**
5. **Discoloration and abnormal pigmentation**
6. **Deepening nasolabial line or fold from corners of nostrils to corners of mouth**
7. **Parenthesis-like lines at corners of mouth**
8. **Vertical frown lines between eyebrows**
9. **Superficial lines in upper lip**
10. **Slight fullness along jawline, causing loss of clean, straight look**
11. **Fullness under jaw**
12. **Small fatty pouches alongside mouth**

These are all simple problems, which, as you will see, can be easily prevented or corrected. Untreated, they increase exponentially until only surgical intervention will help.

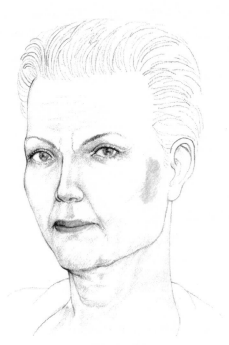

Later stages of changes as listed below.

1. **Excess skin of upper eyelids, puffiness under eyes**
2. **Nasolabial folds fully developed and line etched in skin**
3. **Vertical lines in lip becoming permanent crevasses**
4. **Deepening vertical lines between eyebrows**
5. **Jowls developing over jawline**
6. **Hanging skin and deep wrinkles**

How discouraging. Magnified and compressed, this is reality. The following chapters will help you understand how we intend to stop all these changes before they take hold.

tools of
THE TRADE

[ALPHA HYDROXY ACID PEELS]

A lpha hydroxy acid is everywhere. Some preparations call it fruit acid; others combine the names with proprietary products. The active ingredients remain the same. The difference between medical alpha hydroxy acid treatments and over-the-counter preparations is the concentration of the active ingredients and the vehicle in which they are delivered. The purpose of the preparations is to exfoliate the dead cell layer of the stratum corneum, encourage growth of new cells, and eliminate superficial wrinkles and discolorations. They seem to have a positive effect on the nature of collagen as well. The preparations are available in various strengths and are reasonably effective. Under controlled circumstances what is produced is not quite a peel; nor are the side effects and possible complications of true peels associated with it. The objective is a turnover of the superficial layer of skin without the deep peel component that causes redness, flaking, and swelling in deep peels.

This is the very same preparation available over-the-counter under so many trade names. The strength of the commercial preparations is unregulated by law, but it rarely exceeds 10 percent, which makes them very safe for long-term treatment and maintenence. Medical preparations of the same material contain up to 70 percent alpha hydroxy acid and are quite effective. The usual course of treatment for early skin changes, discolorations, and fine wrinkles is a series of office visits at which increasingly strong solutions are used. The alpha hydroxy acid is painted on the skin and left in place for several minutes until a tingling sensation is felt. At that point the solution is washed off with cold water. The tingling stops, and the skin may look red for up to a few hours. There is no actual peeling though some skin flakes off over the postpeel period. The patient applies a mild AHA preparation nightly to keep up the low-level acid activity, and the cycle is repeated every two weeks for six sessions.

The effect of these treatments is cumulative, due to both the increasing strength of the solution used and the repetition of the process. Positive changes are noticed by virtually all patients and the risks are very minimal. An occasional individual may react to the strong solution with a sunburn-like effect, but that is fleeting. Transient discoloration has been reported, but that is usually resolved as well. The rare cases of persistent discoloration respond well to treatment with bleaching agents. The overall result is smoother, more lustrous skin, free of discoloration, blemishes, irregularities of the surface, and fine wrinkles. This is a treatment I suggest to most patients thirty and over. It works well at cleaning, revitalizing, and rejuvenating the skin, and should be part of a biannual routine. As the need for treatment increases, more concentrated solutions are used. Most often the skin is prepared with tretinoin for several weeks prior to peel. That not only seems to make the peel more effective; it also promotes more rapid healing.

As discussed in the section on over-the-counter preparations, you can actually benefit from the over-the-counter preparations of AHA, as well. They are particularly good for maintaining the status quo after other treatments, and these less concentrated preparations are a good periodic exfoliant for younger people. They are safe and the results are visible. Nevertheless, most other over-the-counter preparations are required by law to be largely ineffective. All the hype one sees about the efficacy of each new product changing the nature of the skin, initiating great biochemical changes, or renewing collagen are pretty much nonsense. If these preparations entered the substance of the skin rather than affecting only the dead cells on the surface, they would be classified as drugs, undergo the scrutiny of the FDA, and, if they actually worked, require a prescription. The irony of the position of the alpha hydroxy acids is that they are not meant to enter the skin. They do their work on the surface, and the limited strength in which they are available over-the-counter or at skin care salons protects the consumer from the dangers of too concentrated an acid peel in unqualified hands, yours or others'. This disclaimer aside, they do work. I usually suggest the medical-grade course to get the skin cleaned up and healthy looking, and salon or commercial preparations for routine maintenance.

Since these treatments do not require anesthesia, they are usually performed by the nursing staff, under the doctor's supervision. Fees are fairly modest and currently tend to range between $100 and $300 per session. Six sessions, two weeks apart, are recommended for maximum benefit.

[TRETINOIN]

This is a subject that seems to interest everyone. Tretinoin is the generic name for the active ingredient of Retin-A, the trade name for the pioneering product produced by the Ortho Pharmaceutical Corporation. It has become a part of the beauty jargon. Other products also contain tretinoin, and it is very likely that related compounds will surface under various trade names. Therefore, it makes sense to deal with generic names for active ingredients whenever possible.

Every day there is new information, more promise, and some controversy. The product itself has been around for many years for the treatment of acne. It is a derivative of vitamin A and has properties that cause the skin cells to turn over in a manner that suggests youthful behavior. With regular usage the outer, visible, keratinized layer becomes smoother and less irregular, some blemishes disappear, and fine wrinkles diminish. Recent work indicates that tretinoin actually increases the ability of the skin to produce and lay down collagen within the dermis.

It is generally agreed that all this occurs to some degree. The argument centers on whom it helps and how much. Not surprisingly, the subject is extremely subjective. How bad is a wrinkle? How much does it improve over how long? Does the improvement last? Each individual becomes an isolated judge of progress without close scrutiny or scientific control. There have been numerous reports of great efficacy, some supported by research grants from the Ortho Pharmaceutical Corporation, which produces tretinoin, and others from unaffiliated investigators. A 1996 study even reported that tretinoin usage prior to sun exposure actually controls the activity of enzymes that would otherwise break down collagen and elastin fibers in the skin. In other words, tretinoin would prevent skin damage and wrinkling due to sun exposure. Heavy stuff, indeed. Little has been said of the effects upon the tendency to skin cancer, although it seems to erase some types of precancerous lesions.

Whether all this is true or not, we are surely on the right track. The fact that the product, in a slightly less irritating form, has been cleared for market by the FDA specifically for treatment of wrinkles speaks volumes. Here is the first open approval by this cautious government agency of a product for the purpose of wrinkle treatment. It means the claims of efficacy are not crazy and the product does work. It does not mean it will work for everyone. Intrinsic to the mode of work is an irritating effect on the skin. Some people are unable to cope with the red, scaly surface that develops. It usually abates, but many must discontinue usage because of it. For some the irritation increases with usage and they, too, must abandon therapy. Others use the product for months without visible change. That would be enough to advise abandoning the course if the recent studies didn't offer hope that sun damage can be prevented or perhaps reversed with tretinoin. Could those protective effects be worthwhile enough even though there was no outward improvement? Very possibly. There is too much promise here to abandon usage unless one must. The downside appears minimal and the opportunity seems too good to pass up. Perhaps something better will come along, but do you have ten years to waste waiting? Here is something that holds great promise. If it is not up to the hype, you have lost little.

Tretinoin therapy is begun with 0.25 percent cream. That is the weakest strength available. It is applied nightly to dry skin twenty minutes after proper cleansing, preferably with a mild soap. It is applied thinly in an invisible layer. The original preparation was exceedingly drying; Renova, the new formulation of the drug (and it is a drug), is said to be less so, and therefore less irritating. This would be advantageous to those unable to tolerate the irritation caused by the original formulation. For effects to be visible, the treatment must continue for at least four months. Often increasingly higher-strength creams are used until the level of tolerance is reached. During and for a period of time after treatment, the skin is increasingly sensitive to sun exposure and must be protected by sunscreen. If that is not scrupulously adhered to, blotchy pigmentation may result.

It is not entirely understood whether the use of tretinoin needs to become a permanent part of a long-term routine to achieve and maintain maximal results. It seems wise to allow the skin time to recover from the treatment. Others advise that the effectiveness is based on forcing the skin into more youthful behavior patterns, and therefore should be continual. There is significant overlap in the effect of tretinoin and the alpha hydroxy acids upon wrinkles, skin pigmentation and blemishes, irregularities of the skin surface, and the quality and quantity of the collagen and elastin within the dermis. Additional overlap is provided by the finding that skin treated with tretinoin after peeling heals faster, and skin treated with tretinoin prior to AHA and trichloroacetic acid peels exhibits greater improvement. The balance between these two modalities is still unclear, but both are very important for skin maintenance and treatment.

Tretinoin is perhaps the least invasive of the physician-regulated therapies. It actually straddles a fine line, since it is prescription controlled but patient applied and self-evaluated and -regulated. As the fund of knowledge concerning tretinoin grows, other products will appear, new forms will evolve, and ultimately it will slip into the domain of over-the-counter treatments. It is still necessary to purchase these products from pharmacies with doctors' prescriptions. Your dermatologist or plastic surgeon should play some role in monitoring your progress, and periodic visits after the initial three months are in order; also, the strength of the cream or its frequency of application may be altered. Once these variables are determined, long-term therapy is usually well tolerated.

For now, tretinoin (Retin-A, Renova), should be a part of the treatment and prevention regimen for everyone concerned with youth maintenance.

[BLEACHING CREAMS]

Melanin is the substance responsible for pigment in the skin. Obviously, shades vary among ethnic groups and are genetically determined. Irregular areas of pigmentation break the continuum of coloration, and catch the eye. For fair-skinned individuals in particular, these areas of darker skin contrast sharply with the basic coloration. The pigmented areas may take any of a number of forms, most of which are unattractive, and most of which are of no true medical significance. For many of these problems, there are reasonably effective methods to control excess pigmentation.

However, little progress has been made in the treatment of pigment-depletion problems. They may take the form of spontaneous pigment loss, called vitiligo, or be the result of peels, dermabrasion, or other medical treatments. Hyperpigmentation, the accumulation of excess pigment, has many known causes as well. They include sun exposure, response to medications such as birth control pills, surgery, and aging.

The simplest and most effective treatment for hyperpigmentation is the use of bleaching creams. Bleaching creams work by inhibiting the enzyme tyrosinase, which is necessary for the production of melanin, and hence pigment. The most frequently used products are based on the compound hydroquinone, which performs this function. Application of hydroquinone to dark spots causes the keratinocytes in the skin to reduce melanin production. That takes at least four weeks to show results, since the old hyperpigmented cells must be shed before the new, lighter cells surface. So bleaching agent is a misnomer. Nothing is bleached, but the new crop of skin cells are less pigmented, and the dark areas recede.

Hydroquinone is prescription regulated in its effective 3 percent and 4 percent strength, and is provided in many forms. The various options should be discussed with a physician. While using this therapy, sun exposure must be avoided. That can be done by avoidance or sunscreen, or both. Sunlight is self-defeating as it promotes pigmentation. Some manufacturers deal with this by adding sunscreen to the hydroquinone preparation.

Irregular areas of hyperpigmentation are far more common a problem than one would imagine. It is more prevalent in women due to the ubiquitous nature of birth control pills and pregnancy, both of which are primary causes of this phenomenon. Other drug reactions and sun exposure account for much of the incidence. For others, the naturally occurring dark under-eye circles qualify, while other individuals have age-related sunspots. In all but the most glaring situations, women tend to cover the areas with makeup, and men tend to ignore them alto-gether. The availability of effective treatment has begun to offer hope. In some situations, superficial peels help relieve the problem, but the first line of defense should be bleaching creams and sunblock. Currently, hydroquinone is the only easily managed, reliable *bleaching* agent available.

Areas of reduced or absent pigment present a more difficult problem, and one for which there is no easy and effective solution.

[COLLAGEN]

Collagen comprises the substance of the skin. Its loss causes inelasticity, sag-ging, and wrinkling, so naturally it would seem worthwhile to try to replace the loss. The search for the perfect replacement material has been going on for decades. The closest scientists have come is the replacement of human collagen with the purified version of bovine collagen. The most popular form is called Zyplast. It is produced by the Collagen Corporation, from collagen recovered from bovine skin. As with any foreign substance, there is great concern over the possibility of allergy to the injected matter. Fortunately, the actual proteins com-prising cow collagen are very similar to ours and are very well tolerated; hence, the incidence of allergy is very small. The possibility of allergy is tested for by a small subcutaneous skin injection in the forearm. Immediate and late allergy are known to occur, and a waiting period of three weeks is advised before starting treatments. Even in the face of negative skin tests, allergy can develop. The red-ness, swelling, and discoloration that occur usually resolve in six to twelve weeks. Drugs can help, but the experience is unpleasant and, happily, rare. Reports of more serious problems such as autoimmune reactions are periodically reported, but not clearly proven. The millions of collagen injections given over the years have proven very safe. I have seen only one serious allergic reaction, and as luck

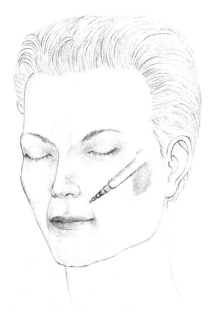

Collagen is effective, if temporary, treatment for nasolabial folds, lip lines, and vertical frown lines.

would have it, the patient was a movie star who was referred to me red and swollen during the making of a film. She had been successfully using collagen for touch-up before shooting for years when she became allergic. The problem took months to subside and the lady in question was furious when I refused to treat her with collagen a year later.

For the most part, the good news about collagen is that bad results or bad reactions don't persist; the bad news is that good results are temporary as well. The body metabolizes and breaks down the injected collagen at varying rates. A life span of less than six months is average. The collagen is provided in a gel form and is injected superficially with a very fine needle. Each pinprick stings a bit, but a small amount of anesthetic in the mix dulls the area for repeat injections. To keep it in perspective, everyone complains a bit of the discomfort, and everyone comes back for more, because it works.

The concept is to fill wrinkles and small skin folds with collagen in order to reduce their depth and temporarily relieve them. The most successfully treated areas are the vertical frown lines between the eyebrows, the nasolabial lines, and the fine lines about the lips and corners of the mouth. All these areas can be treated in a single session, usually with a 1.0- or 1.5-cubic-centimeter (cc) dose. The injections appear reddened like mosquito bites for a short while after treatment. That subsides in an hour or two. The treatment need not alter your schedule. Most people return to normal activities immediately after treatment. Collagen is also used to plump out the lips. That usually requires a slightly larger volume and often results in a day or two of swelling because of the great vascularity of the lips. Not at all unlike the reaction to trauma in the area.

The cost of collagen treatments is usually based upon the amount used. It is provided in individual tubes of 1.0 and 1.5 cc, and fees range between $300 and $500 per dose. This can become expensive when the effect dissipates quickly. If the same area requires treatment more often than two or three times a year, one should rethink the use of collagen.

[FIBREL]

Fibrel is another substance available to fill in wrinkles. Like collagen, its effects are temporary, though an infrastructure of connective tissue is said to persist after the material itself dissipates, giving a longer-lasting result. A gelatin substance is mixed with one's own blood and the mixture reinjected into the wrinkle or depression. The injection hurts a bit more than collagen, I have been told. There is minimal allergy reported with Fibrel, and it may last longer than collagen, but there seem to be few other advantages. Collagen is simpler, more easily tolerated, and far more popular. Most of us have little or no experience with Fibrel, and nothing I have heard makes me wish to reconsider.

[DEEP SKIN PEELS]

Deep skin peels include a small range of options. I tend to use the term to differentiate the category from the "superficial peels," such as the alpha hydroxy acid peels discussed earlier. The deep peels are obviously more aggressive, and are designed to work more deeply into the skin in an effort to eliminate wrinkles. But before you jump to the conclusion that deeper is better, you need to know something about the reality of the use of peels.

The concept of deep skin peeling is to remove the damaged and denatured collagen of the skin and replace it with a smoother and healthier version. This actually works. It not only eliminates wrinkles, but produces tighter, more elastic skin. As late as 1975, the only peeling agent being widely used was a phenol-based solution. This is a very caustic agent that essentially dissolves the epidermis and superficial dermis, taking along with the cellular debris both superficial and deep wrinkles. The actual mechanism of healing produces good, thick bands of elastic collagen in the dermis that are far stronger and healthier than the collagen present before peeling. In this manner the skin becomes rejuvenated, better looking, and more resilient.

Being quite effective, the phenol peel should be a most useful tool. Unfortunately, the depth of peel is difficult to control, and is associated with a whole list of complications. Some of these complications are technical and uncommon; others are far more frequently seen. Most often encountered is a loss of pigmentation in the peeled area. Therefore, the line of demarcation between peeled and unpeeled areas is sometimes sharp and noticeable. Often the phenol-peeled area is covered with a mask of impermeable tape or ointment, to increase the efficacy of the chemicals. This area is not only out of our control, but is also out of sight. Think about treating the vertical lines about the lips with this peel. The area is cleansed, the phenol applied, and the area covered with tape or an occlusive ointment. If the treatment is effective, there is the risk of the entire area around the mouth being bleached of color, contrasting sharply with the untreated areas. Some practitioners avoid this line of demarcation by treating the entire face. Unfortunately, the line of peel has to end somewhere. The color line may be at the jawline or the neck, or perhaps there will be no change in color at all. The point is, the procedure is unpredictable. Even if this problem doesn't occur, and in the majority of cases it doesn't, there remains the slim chance of deep burn and scarring, or, if sun exposure is resumed in the healing phase, of dark, splotchy discoloration. Phenol peels have occasionally been associated with cardiac arrhythmias, and therefore must be performed under carefully monitored circumstances.

The phenol peel presents a delicate balance in trying to achieve the desired effect while avoiding complications. Still, there was a time when we all used phenol peels, simply because there were no viable alternatives. It was the best and most popular treatment for facial wrinkles. Patients accepted risks, few had significant problems, and besides, it was all we had to offer. Happily, that is no longer the case. With the advent of more superficial peeling agents, particularly when combined with other ingredients, we are able to achieve better results in a safer, more controlled environment. But don't be lulled into thinking the newer peels are risk-free. They are not risk-free, but they are considerably safer than phenol. Here I am referring only to the trichloroacetic acid (TCA) peel. Not the more superficial, and very safe, alpha hydroxy acid treatments, which are dealt with at great length elsewhere.

Having said all this, there remains a place for phenol peels. Many plastic surgeons and dermatologists swear by them, and get very good results. I personally believe the risk/reward ratio is too high, particularly with so many other effective tools available.

One of those very effective methods is TCA. Here again, the procedure is not risk-free. It is easier to manage TCA peels and they are considerably safer than phenol peels, but they are not risk-free. The major upside is that the TCA peels produce less color loss than phenol, and by their nature, can be varied in concentration for application to different problem areas of the face. That is important since skin thickness varies considerably in different locations. The areas around the eyes and eyelids have very fine, thin skin; therefore, one can safely use weaker concentrations of TCA to revitalize those areas. This sort of tailoring of the concentration of the agent is not possible with phenol.

Patients are often routinely pretreated with Retin-A and a bleaching agent prior to TCA peels. This seems to enhance efficacy and promote rapid healing. As with all deep peels, the procedure is performed under well-monitored conditions, and usually with the patient sedated. These are not procedures for home use or the beauty salon.

As far as the patient is concerned, there a significant upside to the TCA peel, at least compared with phenol. First of all, the postpeel period is significantly less hideous. True, the skin swells, but not nearly as much. A brownish layer of dead skin develops, which is covered by ointment and separates with washing. New skin appears in less than a week, and makeup can then be used to cover the pink cast that persists for some weeks. All in all, it is a quicker and less traumatic experience. That's the good news. The bad news is that phenol usually does a better and longer-lasting job on the very deep wrinkles. But, on balance, TCA seems to be the peel of choice for facial wrinkles and blemishes. The results are uniformly good, the risk of discoloration or excessively deep peeling is reduced, and both the procedure and recovery are more easily tolerated.

Each of the three types of therapeutic peel has its use. The phenol peel still seems to be the most effective in treating long-standing deep wrinkles. The downside is a higher incidence of complications and a longer healing period. TCA peels are nearly as effective as phenol, excellent for slightly less deep wrinkles, and offers the benefits of fewer complications and faster recovery. AHA peels are more superficial still and must be performed in a series of treatments. Even then, they are not useful for the treatment of deep wrinkles. AHA is very well tolerated and virtually complication-free, but is reserved for the treatment of fine wrinkles, discolorations and irregularities, and overall improvement of the condition and appearance of the skin.

It is hard to predict how long after peeling wrinkles reappear. That is a function of individual skin and lifestyle, just as the original wrinkles are. The cost of these treatments varies from $200 for each AHA peel, to $2,000 or $3,000 or more for the deeper peels, depending on how large an area is treated, whether anesthesia is necessary, and other variables.

[DERMABRASION]

This is an old and much maligned tool. Before the wide array of peels currently available, before collagen, and before the laser, dermabrasion and phenol peeling were the only choices for treating wrinkles. Used properly, and for proper indications, it works quite well, but the list of indications has shrunken greatly.

The procedure is nothing more than applying a rotating burr or metal brush to the skin. As you might imagine, the result is not pretty. The top layer of the skin is removed and the dermis is entered, in the hope that the regenerated skin will be smooth and taut. Meanwhile, the patient looks like she slid into third base on her face. The next ten days are spent nursing the wounds and waiting for enough healing to allow application of makeup to mask the angry pink skin, which gradually returns to normal color over the weeks. The technique has been reasonably successful in treating acne scarring. Far from perfect, but good enough to warrant the trouble, though most practitioners have abandoned it in favor of the carbon dioxide laser even for this application.

Dermabrasion is also helpful in dealing with small areas of deep wrinkles. Unfortunately, the spinning wheel makes it difficult to evaluate depth and uniformity. Here, too, it has been largely abandoned in favor of the more controllable laser. The long-term improvement in collagen alignment and density does not equal that achieved with peeling, and here again dermabrasion has fallen from favor.

For our purposes, dermabrasion is important primarily for its conceptual value; introducing the idea of mechanical resurfacing of the skin. It still finds application in the treatment of an isolated wrinkle or depression in the skin. From personal communication with other plastic surgeons, I can confidently say that those of us who have access to a carbon dioxide laser no longer use dermabrasion. The cost of dermabrasion depends upon the size of the area treated, and can vary from several hundred to several thousand dollars.

[LASER WRINKLE REMOVAL]

The newest treatment for surface wrinkles is CO_2 laser resurfacing. Lasers, the acronym for light amplification by stimulated emission of radiation, are focused high-energy light waves whose force is harnessed and finely directed by an integrated computer. Over the years various types of lasers have been used in surgery. Most recently the CO_2 laser has been fitted with a pulsed control that allows it to deliver rapid and concentrated beams of light to the skin. The computer allows the depth of penetration to be accurately controlled. The pattern coursed over a wrinkled skin area results in skin destruction to the level of the papillary dermis. This effectively wipes out the layer of skin containing the wrinkles, while preserving the layer necessary for skin regeneration. The speed and accuracy of the procedure has made it an immensely popular tool. Theoretically, dermabrasion or deep chemical peel should be equally effective in wrinkle ablation, but the reality is different. Depth of treatment cannot be accurately gauged other than with the computerized laser. It is the only treatment performed at the appropriate and uniform depth throughout. That allows for aggressive accuracy without worry of overly deep penetration. It is particularly valuable for treating specific wrinkles such as vertical lip lines or the thin skin of the lower eyelid, as well as for full-face resurfacing. There appear to be superior results with far fewer side effects.

The laser procedure is performed in the doctor's office. Both plastic surgeons and dermatologists offer the service. The area to be treated is injected with a local anesthetic and the laser is patterned on the skin in a series of narrowly separated dots. This superficial layer of coagulated skin is wiped away with a moist gauze pad and a second pass is made over or alongside the actual deep wrinkle. This, too, is wiped away and an ointment is applied. The area is kept clean and moist, and new pink skin covers the treated area in about a week. At that point, cosmetics can be used for coverage. Eight to twelve weeks will pass before normal skin color returns.

The areas where the CO_2 laser has proven invaluable to me are the difficult to treat vertical lines in the upper lip, furrows at the corners of the mouth, lower face and chin wrinkles, and smile lines. Total facial resurfacing with the CO_2 laser is also easily tolerated and quite effective.

Wrinkle treatment and resurfacing seem the best application for the CO_2 laser, though it is sold and promoted as a substitute for the surgical scalpel. True, it can cut through tissue, but it does so very slowly compared with traditional surgery and offers no discernible advantage. The key to the reality of this situation is reflected in the promoters of this use, primarily nonplastic surgeons with no training in complex procedures such as eye-lift and face-lift, offering "bloodless laser surgery." Qualified plastic surgeons have generally shunned the use of the laser for cosmetic surgery and restricted its use to wrinkle ablation and skin resurfacing, where it excels. In fact, the use of the CO_2 laser has generally supplanted both deep peels and dermabrasion for the treatment of specific problems such as perioral (around the mouth) wrinkles and smile lines. Those physicians who have access to the laser swear by it. For use over greater areas such as full-face resurfacing, there has been some resistance to laser usage, since TCA peels have long been effective, are quickly performed, are less costly, and offer a shorter recovery period. These are obviously important considerations, but the results using the laser are generally superior. This, however, remains an area of controversy.

In many ways the argument is self-serving. Those physicians who have made an investment of some \$100,000 in the CO_2 laser love it. Those who have had little or no experience with the laser, and haven't made the investment, feel it is unnecessary. True, we did get along without it for all those years, but much the same comment can be made about most advances. Laser technology and the results of wrinkle ablation and skin resurfacing are a great step forward.

The cost of all this new technology is usually greater than for the other options. A perioral TCA or phenol peel to remove wrinkles of the lips, chin, and corners of the mouth can generally cost between \$500 and \$1,000. Laser treatment of the same area could cost twice that, but the result justifies the expense.

[MICROSUCTION]

Here is a wonderfully effective and minimally invasive new technique. Before I try to wiggle my way out of whether microsuction is invasive, let me tell you what it means, and what it does. *Microsuction* is a term I began using some years ago to describe liposuction, using tiny specialized instruments for the treatment of particular facial problems. As you doubtless know, liposuction refers to the surgical removal of fat using a vacuum apparatus and sterile steel tubes that look something like drinking straws. Carrying that analogy further, the straws come in varied lengths and calibers, depending on the task to be performed. The usual diameter for body liposuction is between 4 to 5 millimeters, or nearly one quarter of an inch. In microsuction the catheter is 1 to 2 millimeters, a very fine instrument for the controlled removal of limited amounts of fat in special areas about the face. The procedure was devised to deal with the tiny fat pouches that tend to develop alongside the corners of the mouth, the small accumulations of fat along the jawline and neck, and the folds that develop along the nasolabial line from the corners of the nose to the corners of the mouth. Removing the fatty spots helps a lot, of course, but as a side benefit the microsuction irritates the undersurface of the skin and seems to stimulate it to tighten and look better.

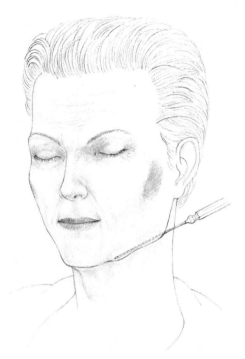

Fine microsuction catheter inserted behind earlobe and passed along jawline to treat jowls.

Another area where this does wonders is the double chin. Doing this procedure for people with all levels of the problem has had very impressive results both for the new angularity and the obvious tightening effect on the skin. The effect has been so good that in many cases it can eliminate the need for neck-lift. But of course, that is the extreme example. More often, this procedure is best for smaller areas and for individuals in their early forties, whose skin retains healthy elasticity. The sum of all this is that if the fatty accumulations along the jaw, and elsewhere, are dealt with early by microsuction, not only are they eliminated, but the skin over them tightens and adds to the result. Here the sum is greater than its parts.

Often simply inserting the finest catheter from behind the earlobe, along the jawline, is all that is necessary to correct and tighten early loosening of the jawline. This is a minor procedure that delivers a quick, refreshing correction. It is not a substitute for surgery but sometimes is all that is necessary to deal with a particular situation. Simple microsuction of the jawline and the pouches alongside the mouth should be considered whenever a patient is undergoing eyelid or other facial surgery. It is a disservice not to think of it, for so much can be gained so easily. The addition of microsuction of the jawline or mouth adds little to the operative time, and nothing to recovery time.

Microsuction is performed under local anesthesia, with or without sedation. A tiny hole is made either under the chin or behind the earlobes, through which the microsuction catheter is introduced. These sites are chosen because they make for easy access to the trouble spots, and they are not readily visible. The result of the procedure is immediately visible, though masked a bit by swelling over a week or two. In general, you look better than before microsuction as soon as whatever bruising has occurred recedes. The actual result matures over six or eight weeks. At that point all the swelling has gone and the skin is as taut as it is going to be. The procedure is very, very low-risk. I know better than to say that any procedure is risk-free, but if I were forced to pick one, this would probably be it. The major downside is that perhaps an individual, for whatever reason, doesn't have as impressive a result as anticipated. There also may be injury to a nerve, from injection or the procedure itself. This is an exceedingly rare event and is usually self-limiting. That is certainly a disappointment.

In general, this simple procedure takes about twenty minutes to do, and effectively removes some of the earmarks of early aging, smooths the lower-face contours, and tightens the skin. All this without traditional surgery, and with minimal recovery time and little or no risk. Sounds too good to be true, but for the appropriate patients it buys years of good looks, and pushes the need for surgery years down the road. The cost for facial microsuction varies from $1,000 to $3,000, depending on the extent of treatment and whether it is being combined with other procedures.

[LIPOSUCTION]

Liposuction, or suction-assisted lipectomy, as it seems to be officially called, is the world's most frequently performed cosmetic surgery procedure. Everyone knows about it and everyone talks about it, and all this in just over ten years. That is long enough for it to have fallen out of fashion had the procedure not lived up to its hype. An astounding ascent out of nowhere to a permanent place in the public perception of plastic surgery.

It remains unclear when the procedure originated, but it was popularized in France, in the late 1970s and early '80s. Since then, popularity of liposuction has taken off. Why? Because it works, and the result is permanent!

The procedure is based conceptually on the fact that there are finite numbers of fat cells per square inch of tissue. For the sake of example, say 100 cells per square inch. These individual cells have the ability to enlarge and shrink according to the fluctuations of body weight and individual genetic predisposition, but they do not increase in number. Assume that instead of the 100 cells per square inch you might have generally throughout your body, there are 150 cells per square inch around your hips. Since the number of cells is fixed, there are more cells to enlarge in the area around your hips than the rest of your body. As you gain weight, you will gain half again as much in that area as in the surrounding tissue with fewer cells per square inch. If you lose weight, all the cells in your body will get smaller. There are more cells per square inch around your hips. Each cell will be reduced in size, but because of the larger number of cells, the area will continue to be out of proportion. If the extra fat cells were removed by liposuction, the area would then look proportional, and you would gain or lose weight in a more symmetrical manner. Those extra fat cells that were removed would not return. You could certainly gain weight, and some of that weight would return to the treated areas, but in proportion to the weight gain in the rest of your body. The saddlebag hips would not return.

The thrust of the discussion thus far should have interested you, but it is clearly applicable to large areas of the body, not the face, and is seemingly not related to the Youth Corridor. After all, this is a genetically determined problem that crosses generational borders. True, all true. But the face is not excluded from these problems, and aging changes the redistribution of fat in the subcutaneous tissue of the face. The instruments used in liposuction of the body have been altered specifically, in scale and delicacy, for facial use, and the process has become increasingly useful. For example, the double chin was previously treated by surgical fat removal through a fairly large incision. The results were uneven at best. Now, with microsuction, a tiny catheter is introduced through a quarter-inch incision under the chin and the fat can be easily removed, resulting in complete reversal of the problem, and a smooth and much tighter neck and jawline.

The procedure has been further refined to deal with the accumulation of fatty pockets on the face resulting from multiple causes, including gravity and loss of elasticity of the skin. Much of the more delicate work falls into the microsuction category. This differs in several ways from the general category of liposuction. First, the size of the catheter used in microsuction is of the finest caliber for the delicate process of removing small fat deposits. Second, in liposuction one intentionally leaves a uniform layer of fat attached to the undersurface of the skin. That allows a smooth and dimple-free result. In microsuction, the fat is removed from the undersurface of the skin, and the skin itself is abraded with the catheter. This seems to encourage contraction of the delicate facial skin. These, and other purely technical factors, lead me to categorize microsuction separately from the larger family of liposuction. Based on the same theory, both are enormously important and successful tools.

[CORRUGATOR RESECTION]

The corrugators are a pair of tiny muscles that really leave their mark. These small bands are part of the muscles of facial expression. They originate at

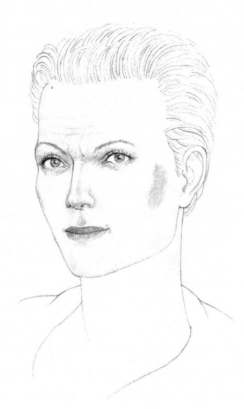

Vertical frown lines between the eyebrows caused by the action of the corrugator muscles.

the bony rim beneath the eyebrows, and course horizontally to insert into the skin between the eyebrows over the bridge of the nose. When one is relaxed, they relax and there is no sign of them, or what they do. When one frowns or makes quizzical expressions, these little devils snap into action. They are the muscles that contract, draw the skin between the eyebrows together, and form the vertical furrows above the bridge of the nose. Everyone has them, and everyone can produce those furrows. Some of us have more active corrugator muscles, frown more frequently, and produce permanent vertical lines etched into the skin between the eyebrows. Again, the repetitive action ultimately etches the frown lines into the skin. This kind of action is a form of tensing the facial muscles, and again you can see how facial muscle exercises can lead to wrinkles. These are among the earliest appearing deep facial wrinkles, and often stand conspicuously against an otherwise unlined forehead. They have the ability to impart a strained, tense countenance, and are never flattering. Happily, there is a simple, effective, and permanent treatment.

Since the corrugator muscles serve only to produce those frown lines, and since other related muscles can continue to animate the brow, eliminating the corrugators would be no loss, and considerable gain. That is exactly what we do. Cutting the muscles eliminates the majority of the vertical frown lines, smooths the brow, and prevents the development of further lines. This has proven to be a simple, effective procedure, and should be considered when one notices the gradual etching of these frown lines into the skin. The earlier the lines are dealt with, the better and more complete the result.

Corrugator muscle resection is performed under local anesthesia and a bit of sedation. I usually suggest the sedation because people get anxious about someone fussing so near their eyes. A small incision is made in the natural skin fold of the upper lid, close to the nose. The length of the incision is about half an inch, and soon becomes virtually invisible. If the patient is having her eyes done, the corrugator procedure is performed at the same time, through the same upper-lid incision. It adds little extra time and no further discomfort to the procedure. The thin corrugator muscle is easily identified and a tiny section is cut across it. The wound heals in a few days and patients report no difficulty with expression. The vertical lines between the brows are greatly reduced or eliminated, and while collagen injections or fat transplants may be necessary to iron out long-standing lines, the muscle resection will prevent a new crop.

This is a very nice tool, since there is great physical improvement from so small a procedure. Something about a permanent scowl, or even the lines that suggest it, detracts greatly from an attractive face. This procedure can be the answer. Costs vary from $1,000 to $2,500, depending on the surgeon and what other procedures are being performed. Most often, corrugator resection is done with eyelid surgery, but increasingly it is being performed earlier and for younger patients. The object being to control the frowning *before* the vertical lines are etched into the skin.

[BOTOX]

A temporary method to smooth out the same vertical frown lines that corrugator resection corrects, as well as horizontal forehead furrows, is the injection of Botox. Frighteningly enough, this safe substance is produced from botulism toxin, a deadly poison. Though no longer toxic, the substance retains the ability to temporarily paralyze the nerves it surrounds. It is injected near the nerves supplying the corrugators, or other facial muscles, and for a period of time irons out the deep furrows by paralyzing the muscles that cause them. A treatment usually lasts about six months, and the results are immediate and dramatic. Unfortunately, there is always the risk of imbalanced paralysis of one side compared with the other, or perhaps early recovery of one side. This makes for a distorted and unpleasant outcome, requiring reinjection, with effects that may then last longer than side one, and so on. Experienced Botox practitioners and patients claim that this is rare, and are strong supporters of the therapy. It has been used primarily to treat horizontal forehead lines, and the vertical furrows between the eyebrows.

Botox treatments cost several hundred dollars per session. The results are transient, and the costs add up. For areas such as the vertical frown lines between the eyebrows, corrugator resection seems a better alternative. Horizontal forehead folds, however, present a more difficult choice, since the surgical cure requires a forehead-lift, and that is a more extensive procedure. Many people opt for Botox in this situation, until full-facial surgery becomes necessary.

[Fat Transplants]

Fat transplants and fat injections are the same thing. A syringe of fat is removed from one body area, usually where you have more than enough to spare, and transplanted, by injection, to an area that needs to be filled in— usually facial wrinkles or frown lines. Before your imagination runs away with you, here are the ground rules. To begin with, the fat must be transferred from one place to another *on the same individual.* That means that you can't lend or borrow from your friends. There is also the problem of blood supply. The only transplanted fat that survives is that portion that develops a blood supply in its new location, and that requires being in direct contact with the blood vessels of the area. The farther a portion of transplanted fat is from the existing blood vessels, the less likely it is to survive. Without being boringly technical, that severely limits the volume of fat that can be successfully transplanted to an area. You cannot take excess fat from your thighs and enlarge your breasts. Good idea, but it won't work. At least not without microvascular surgery to connect the blood vessels of the fat to the recipient site. Even then, the transplantation of large volumes of fat is unpredictable. It is beyond the scope of this book, and rarely a good idea under any circumstances.

For each of the transplanted fat cells to survive, it must receive a blood supply from the tissue against which it rests. The farther from that living tissue, or the thicker the transplant, the less likely is success. Here we are not talking about inches, but fractions of fractions of an inch. For some tissue to survive this type of free transfer, the maximum is one half of 1 millimeter. Twenty-five millimeters equal 1 inch. Therefore 0.5 mm is equal to one fiftieth of an inch. Not very thick. One can assume fat transplants of at least twice that thickness to survive, since theoretically there is blood supply from both above and below. So, we arrive at one twenty-fifth of an inch, or a bit more. In actual practice, most fat transplants are far thicker than that. That is so for many reasons. First, the caliber of the needle used is fairly large so as not to crush the cells. Then the delivery mechanism is not very precise. Most important, the patient wants that deep line from the corner of the nose to the mouth filled in. So we fill it in. What happens? Well, as you might expect, the line or fold is nicely filled in. It looks great for a few months, but then the line begins to reappear. That happens as the fat that hasn't established a blood supply gets reabsorbed and disappears. Beyond that thin layer that survives, all the fat has served as temporary putty. Not very different from collagen injections, except for that 10 or 20 percent of the fat that will survive permanently. That is a significant step forward. Fat injections, done several times over a period of time, seem to offer at last a partial permanent correction of the defect. Some of this is due to a *take* of the transplanted fat, and some due to a fibrous tissue infrastructure that builds up at the site.

Fat transplants are a simple office procedure performed under a local anesthetic. A fat donor site is chosen, usually the thighs or buttocks. A needle is inserted under local, and a small amount of fat is removed. The site for treatment is prepared with local, a pocket made in the area to receive the transplant, and the fat is injected. The entire procedure takes about twenty minutes. There is little swelling or discoloration, and one can plan on returning to work the next day. It is usually a good idea to slightly overcorrect the area to compensate for swelling and the local anesthetic. Significant overcorrection will make the result last somewhat longer, but looks unnatural.

This is an excellent procedure that offers good results. Unfortunately, many people are being misled about what can actually be accomplished. You cannot pump the nasolabial fold full of fat and get a full and permanent correction. Some will persist, but the overwhelming portion of the fat is no more than temporary putty, and will soon be reabsorbed. That's fine, and not very different from collagen, but understand what to expect. Again, however, what differentiates this from collagen is the fact that no foreign substances are involved, and some 10 to 20 percent of the injected volume may be permanent.

Then there is the question of harvesting large amounts of fat, freezing it, and administering it over time. That makes very little sense, as there is no evidence that the fat cells survive freezing, and therefore the injections are merely filler. Physicians employing frozen fat inject it weekly or monthly and claim a connective tissue buildup at the site. Thus far, there is little objective evidence to support this contention, but at worst one is being treated with a well-tolerated natural filler.

Which lasts longer, fat or collagen? I don't know. Both collagen and injected fat give visible improvement for up to six months, but results vary widely. Over the long run, fat transplants will be better, as a percentage of the fat cells survive. If you stick with it and have the procedure repeated, you will get a significant degree of permanent correction. The cost of fat transplants varies widely, but seems to average between $1,000 and $2,000 per session.

[IMPLANT MATERIALS AND IMPLANTS]

Over the years, there is a natural attrition of collagen in areas of constant movement. This may take the form of deep nasolabial folds in the cheeks, which result from the effects of smiling, chewing, and gravity, or one of many other visible and invisible forms. There are many techniques for correcting these areas, and we have already covered the majority of them, the most common being collagen injections and fat transplants. They fill the defect, but are temporary, and perhaps for that reason, are not considered implants. By the same reasoning, silicone shots, which for better or worse, are permanent, would be considered implants.

There are all sorts of materials currently available as implants. A good many of them are Space Age stuff, some of the rest are old standbys, and all depend for success on creative judgment and good taste. Generally, facial implants are designed to fill in defects and increase proportions. Cheekbone and chin implants augment proportions and are permanent. They are made of Silastic, Proplast, or other well-tolerated substances. Often employed in antiaging surgery, implants can enhance the appearance of the jawline and take up a bit of slack skin. Cheek implants increase angularity, and even aging, wrinkled skin looks better draped over graceful, high cheekbones or a strong chin. Angularity suits our concept of beauty in part because it makes use of highlights and shadows. It accentuates what is good, drawing attention away from the rest. Often when a face-lift is performed, cheekbone implants will be inserted on top of existing natural cheekbones. Those implants add angularity and increase the effect of the surgery. They provide a high point for draping the skin and take up slack.

Some implants are specifically used for tissue replacement, though they may have been designed for other applications, some far removed from medicine. The material used must be tolerated by the body, stable over time, and relatively easy to use. Additionally, the material must have been cleared by the FDA for use as a medical substance. Often there is a gray area between FDA clearance and current usage. A good example is Gore-Tex, which is available for use in the United States, but not presently in every applicable form. Gore-Tex fiber strips both fill in wrinkles and increase proportions, are permanent, and have been much publicized for a variety of interesting applications. This is the same material lining your coat and shoes. It has numerous useful properties; among them are malleability and maintenance of integrity. The porous nature of the material allows tissue to grow through it and prevent displacement, and the material itself is very inert, allowing the body to accept it readily.

Strips and threads of Gore-Tex have been used as filler for the nasolabial folds and upper-lip augmentation. The nasolabial Gore-Tex implant is used instead of fat transplants or collagen. Its use is not generally applauded by the community of plastic surgeons for a number of reasons, among them the fact that long-term results are not yet available. That is true of all new procedures, but there have been numerous problems specifically related to the implantation of these strips. Among them is visibility of the implant under the skin and irregularities of the surface above the implant. The same can be said for the strip of the material inserted under the skin of the upper lip. In theory this could serve to plump the lip and obliterate vertical lip lines. There have been many excellent results. The idea and the properties of the material all make sense. It is well tolerated, flexible, stays in place, and should be an excellent resource, but there is not much evidence on which to predict long-term results.

The cost of the implant material itself is neglible, but is more a function of the surgeons' time.

[BLEPHAROPLASTY]

Blepharoplasty is a fancy medical term for having your eyes done: from *bleph,* pertaining to the eyelids, and *plasty,* to mold. To mold the eyelids! Actually, that might be a very genteel way of describing the procedure, for in reality it amounts to surgically removing the excess skin on and about the lids, and reducing fat pads, which cause baggy eyes.

Blepharoplasty is an astoundingly popular procedure, performed several hundred thousand times yearly in the United States. The fact that the result of the surgery is usually wonderful, and the procedure easily tolerated, accounts for the popularity it enjoys. As an antiaging surgical procedure, it is among the earliest performed, typically in the forties, and increasingly earlier. That should come as no surprise since the skin of the eyelids is the thinnest and most delicate of the face. The eyelids provide an actual mirror of the system and swell at the slightest provocation. Here one finds the first signs of allergy, illness, emotional distress, or the results of last night's Chinese food. Repeated cycles of swelling, and the rubbing that unconsciously follows, takes a toll on the elasticity of the eyelids. When the finest tissue is subjected to the most regular abuse, there can be no surprise in its distortion and the breakdown of elasticity. Each smile etches lines on the outside corners of the eyes, as does each squint to block the sun or see off into the distance. But we have to see and we like to smile and the damage piles up.

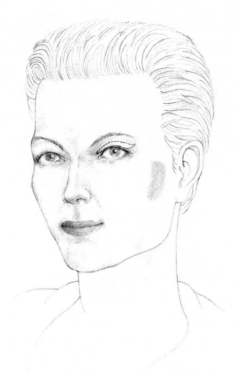

Excess skin of the upper eyelids is marked and removed.

There is a natural loss of elasticity and the eyebrows drop a bit, adding excess tissue to the upper lids. The fat pads of the lower lids become more prominent and bags develop. For some this is congenital; for others it may develop with time. The bags cast a shadow on the ring of skin beneath them, and soon dark circles are added to the brew. At some point in the process, one says, "Enough."

The problem, which took years to develop, takes but an hour to correct. The operation is most often performed in a private clinic or ambulatory surgery facility. It is generally agreed that hospitalization is unnecessary in all but the most unusual circumstances. Intravenous sedation and local anesthetic, usually lidocaine, are all that is necessary. Prior to surgery, the patient's preoperative photographs are studied and compared with her appearance in the recumbent position. We appear suddenly free of the pull of gravity when lying down. When the two realities are integrated, the excess skin of the upper lids is outlined in indelible ink, the patient sedated and local injected to the upper- and lower-lid areas. Marking is not usually necessary on the lower lid, as the incision site is determined by the skin crease just below the lower lashes. The excess skin of the upper lids, which has been marked, is excised along with the tissue beneath it. Fat pockets that cause puffiness of the upper lid are identified and removed. This is particularly important at the inside corner of the eye, where increasing fullness develops over the years. If the patient is at some stage of developing vertical frown lines between the brows, the corrugator muscles that cause the frown are dealt with through the same incision. The upper-lid skin is then closed with a fine nylon suture, which is woven under the skin, to be removed three days later. There are other ways to accomplish this including individual visible sutures or even skin glue. Techniques vary with the common goal of producing a fine and virtually invisible line.

The lower lid is operated through an incision immediately below the lashes, usually in a tiny wrinkle line. It heals rapidly and well, and signs of incision are all but gone within weeks of surgery. After the lower-lid incision is made, a number of variations are possible. One technique is employed if the problem is purely wrinkled skin, another if it is puffiness more than wrinkles. To treat wrinkled skin, the skin itself is separated from the muscle below, the fat pockets are removed through small incisions in the muscle, and the skin is trimmed and redraped in a wrinkle-free, but natural, manner. This is the skin flap technique. If the primary focus is puffiness under the eyes, then the culprit is pockets of excess fat. The muscle beneath the skin is incised without being separated from the skin. This is called a skin-and-muscle flap, and affords excellent access to the fat pockets. The skin and muscle are trimmed and the incision closed with a fine suture.

When the skin-and-muscle flap is employed, the lower-eyelid skin retains its nourishment from the muscle below, and it is safe to perform a peel at the same time. That helps remove fine wrinkles and dark circles below the eyes. When the

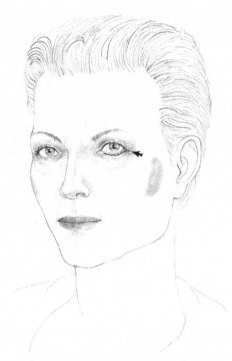

The lower-eyelid incision is made immediately below the eyelashes. No lashes are cut.

situation dictates use of the skin flap technique, peeling is not employed for fear of damaging the already thin skin.

There are any number of complications possible with this surgery. The most common is some degree of dry eye, or alteration in production and quality of tears. This occurs in more than 50 percent of cases and resolves spontaneously. All patients are treated with artificial tears to prevent this discomfort. A more serious, but far less frequent, problem is overaggressive skin removal, which may result in drooping of the lower lid. Other circumstances may cause the same problem, but all are treatable. Excessive upper-lid skin removal can result in an inability to fully close the eyes at rest, but that is usually resolved with time and the pull of gravity, which brings the upper lid down whether we want it to or not.

There are numerous other problems beyond the scope of this brief look, and most are easily dealt with. The best way to avoid problems is knowing they are possible. Having performed thousands of these procedures over the years, it is clear to me that a combination of understanding, experience, and common sense is essential to achieve the best possible result. Hundreds of thousands of blepharoplasties are performed each year, with overwhelmingly good results. It is a popular procedure because it is good and it is safe. The procedure is performed in the office or ambulatory surgery suite and takes about an hour. Heavy sedation and local anesthesia are used and the surgery is very well tolerated. Postsurgical treatment includes twenty-four hours of iced compresses, which control swelling, discoloration, and pain. Most patients don't need analgesics after the first night, if at all. Sutures are removed on the third day. By the end of the week, swelling and discoloration have subsided and eye makeup may be worn. Fees for upper- and lower-lid blepharoplasty range from $3,500 to $7,000.

A properly performed eye-lift, with or without associated procedures, will remove years of wear and tear and restore a lively youth to the central part of your face.

[CLAMPING EYELID WRINKLES]

Another recent addition to the list of little procedures that do a lot, this is the simplest of all eyelid rejuvenators, save peeling, and the quickest fix of all. It is directed at the patient with excess lower-eyelid skin and wrinkles. Not as strange as it sounds. Stand in front of the mirror and smile a few times. If the skin under your eyes doesn't fall back in place, but forms tiny folds and wrinkles, then you see the problem. This is primarily a condition of middle age, though young people with years of sun exposure also exhibit the signs.

The small folds of skin are anesthetized and gently lifted away from the under-

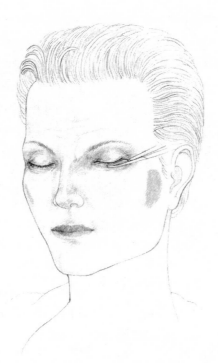

A fine clamp is used to "pinch off" the excess skin of the lower lid.

lying muscle. In proper candidates this is easily done without distorting the eye-lid. A clamp is then used to grasp and compress the excess skin, which is then precisely excised with a fine scissors. There is no bleeding, and the skin is closed with fine sutures that are removed in two or three days. There is virtually no postop swelling or discomfort, and by the end of a week there is little sign of surgery except for the absence of the excess skin.

The skin clamping can be used with any number of other procedures and is often employed as a touch-up for people who have had their eyes done in the past. Complications are rare and recovery is swift. Fees average about $2,000. This is a case of achieving a lot for very little in discomfort and expense.

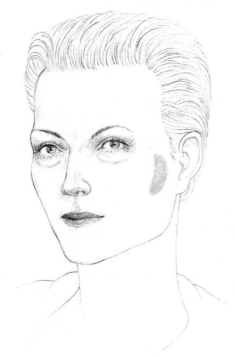

Young people with puffy lower lids are good candidates for subconjuctival blepharoplasty.

[SUBCONJUNCTIVAL BLEPHAROPLASTY]

Another mouthful. Here is an operation restricted to young adults. It treats puffy, baggy lower eyelids in people without loose skin or wrinkles. That lets out all but those in their twenties or thirties who have suffered through youth with people saying, "You look tired. Is anything wrong?" No, there is nothing wrong, and you look tired because you have an inherited excess amount of fat beneath the muscle of your lower lids. It is a family trait. Have a look at the family album. It's there, and it's easy to get rid of.

The term subconjunctival blepharoplasty means that the actual surgery is done through the inner lining of the eyelid and that no visible skin incision is necessary. Under local anesthesia and sedation, the eyelid is held down and the cornea is protected. An incision is made in the eyelid lining, or conjunctiva, in order to reach the fat pockets just deep to the conjunctiva. So the operation is sub, under or deep to, the conjunctiva. After the fat is removed, some ointment may be put over the area and the eye is allowed to close. No sutures are necessary and healing is rapid and invisible. Often some temporary bruising and discoloration result, but otherwise there is no sign of surgery.

The procedure is specifically designed for people with excess fatty bags, but no loose skin or wrinkles. When the fat is removed, the skin becomes less tense, then contracts. If your skin is loose already, or very inelastic, this is not the procedure for you. The ideal patient is young, still unwrinkled, and burdened with unsightly pouches beneath his or her eyes. These people are delighted with the change this small procedure can bring. Fees are in the $2,000 to $4,000 range.

[S-LIFT]

It has always been clear to me, if we are to provide a full range of maintenance options, something must fill the void between simple skin treatments and a full face-lift. As we have already noted, initial facial aging begins on and about the eyelids. Soon after, there begins to develop a generalized, and increasingly noticeable, loss of elasticity, manifested by fleshiness along a formerly clean jawline and deepening of the nasolabial folds. There is loss of cheekbone angularity, some loosening of the skin beneath the neck, or perhaps a bit of a double chin. All this usually happens in the mid-forties, earlier for fine-skinned, fair individuals, later for the thicker-skinned and darker-complexioned. Most notice these changes as the passage from youth. They are not warmly welcomed, nor are they significant enough to elicit thoughts of face-lift. They are too new and not yet overwhelming. A steady despair and resignation sets in, and there seems nothing to do but watch and wait.

Even if a road map of facial wrinkles has not yet appeared, some relief would be welcome. Stop the progress in a young person before the changes have pushed her from youthful to matronly. Clear the jawline and neck, lift the cheekbone prominence to where it used to be, and undo those nasolabial folds along the cheeks and beside the mouth. Yet somehow these simple needs have not been directly addressed.

"Wait, and do a full face-lift when you are ready." That was the advice we offered. None of us, myself included, thought very much of doing less. It wasn't what we were taught and anything less than a full face-lift didn't seem to do the job. Even as the nuances of the surgery and the sophistication of the profession advanced, we held to preconceived notions. It was at this point that I first encountered the rudiments of the S-lift, so named for the lazy S shape of the incision. While I was returning the visits of European colleagues in the early 1980s, one of my hosts demonstrated a procedure that utilized only half of the usual face-lift incision for a far less extensive procedure. The patients got better quickly, and the immediate results were impressive. After ten years of tinkering, only the basic incision remains the same. The new procedure could best be called a two-layer anterior face-lift. It is designed for the earlier stages of facial loosening; it tightens the skin and underlying muscle, effectively lifting everything as in a cradle from under the chin to the forehead. The procedure has become the mainstay in treatment of jowls, cheeks, and forehead, and since we see consistently younger patients who are unwilling to wait for things to get out of hand, my associates and I perform this procedure as often as the traditional face-lift.

Before confusing you any further, we should consider the anatomy of the face, what we are trying to achieve, and the difference between the procedures.

The skin of the face lies on a bed of subcutaneous fat and wispy connective tissue. Except in areas of expression, it is not bound directly to the underlying muscles. That means that there are muscle-skin connections around the eyes, lips and mouth, nose and chin. The entire cheek and neck area, from the ears to the nasolabial fold, is relatively free of firm bonds to the underlying tissues and therefore easily separated and lifted. It also means that these areas are not held firmly in place by any significant bonds to the infrastructure, and are liable to become lax and droop as soon as the skin begins to lose elasticity. That laxity must be corrected, along with the tightening of the underlying muscle fascia, the fine, tough outer coat of the muscle that lends itself to repair. The fascial tightening helps alleviate jowls and deep nasolabial folds and adds longevity to the result. The thin, flat platysma muscle, which lines the skin of the neck, is also tightened to correct the two loose bands under the chin.

The illustration below shows the lazy S incision of the two-layer upper facelift, or S-lift. The hair is combed and held in place with antibiotic ointment. No hair is shaved. The incision arcs across the scalp to the top of the ear, where it is

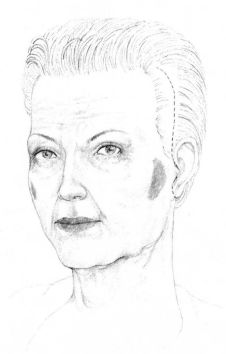

The incision for the S-lift. No hair is shaved.

hidden behind the tragus, that little piece of cartilage that sticks out in front of the ear canal. It then is carried out in front of, and then ends immediately behind, the earlobe. The incision is placed behind the tragus to avoid a telltale scar in front of the ear. The fact that the incision ends at the earlobe means that the unsightly scar behind the ear and along the neck is avoided, which is a great benefit in that you can wear your hair up without fear of exposing what is sometimes a noticeable scar. In fact, there is virtually no visible scar at all. This is a great plus as long as the procedure corrects what must be corrected. The S-lift will not correct a wrinkled or extremely loose neck; nor is it the best procedure to deal with very wrinkled cheeks. These are conditions associated with years of neglected aging or extremely sun-damaged skin. The layered S-lift is designed to correct the loss of elasticity and sagging of early middle age. It provides a good clean look and allows the skin to fit again, without appearing pulled or unnatural. It has become a major factor in maintaining youthful good looks.

The surgery is performed in the private clinic or ambulatory surgery facility under deep sedation and a local anesthetic. Just hearing the word, "local," usually elicits the following statement.

"I don't want to hear anything or feel anything."

Not an unreasonable response, but the level of sedation provided by the anesthesiologist is deep enough for the patient to sleep through the entire procedure. There should be no discomfort and no memory of the procedure itself. More important, the safety level of this sort of anesthesia is excellent. It allows the patient to breathe unassisted and makes the immediate postoperative recovery far smoother than after full general anesthesia, particularly avoiding the need for the endotracheal breathing tube. There is a time and place for general anesthesia, and it should be chosen according to the procedure, patient, and circumstances.

Being ready for an S-lift implies that other changes have likely occurred as well. Unless they have already been done, the S-lift is often performed along with microsuction of the jowls and blepharoplasty. The combined procedure takes just over two hours, after which an additional several hours is spent in the recovery room. Patients are then discharged to home or a recovery facility. Maximum swelling occurs at the third day and rapidly recedes thereafter. There is some bruising, which dissipates after a week, and as a rule patients are able to return to work by the tenth day. The postoperative period is relatively pain-free, complications are few, and recovery is surprisingly swift.

I consider the S-lift the major procedure in the maintenance routine. Even if one follows the routine religiously, there will be progressive loss of elasticity, sagging, and a blunting of facial angles. But the changes will be far less severe and later to appear. For some the procedure may never be necessary at all. Unfortunately, today's adult reader may have arrived late in the skin care revolution; procedures such as the layered S-lift can gracefully undo the damage that has been done.

Fees for this procedure range from $5,000 to $10,000.

[FACE-LIFT]

This is the most serious tool the plastic surgeon has to offer. It comes in many varieties and, except for the incision, has improved greatly over the years. The illustration below shows the hair combed away from the line of incision. Like the S-lift, no hair is shaved, but the incision extends from the forehead scalp to the earlobe. Unlike the modified incision of the S-lift, the incision continues up behind the ear and into the hairline. The operation again lifts the skin from the underlying tissues, but in this case it includes the full face and neck, virtually to the collarbones. Here the operation is designed to deal with more severe skin aging in the form of extensive wrinkling or laxity, hence the greater extent of surgery than with the S-lift. The underlying muscle fascia is tightened, as well as the thin platysma muscle layer of the neck.

The operation is performed in the private clinic or hospital, according to medical needs or patient wishes. The recovery period is a bit longer than for the S-lift and varies between ten days and two weeks. Blepharoplasty and microsuction

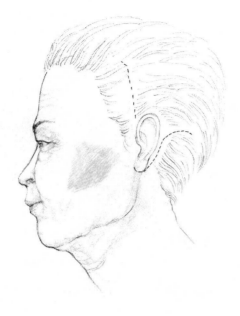

The full face-lift incision.

are usually performed at the same time, and bruising and swelling last the better part of a week. Possible complications of the surgery include hematoma, a collection of blood under the skin that must be drained, and a host of other problems that are usually self-limited or easily corrected. The most dreaded possible complication is injury to the nerve that animates the face. It is a very rare complication, indeed, and most surgeons will not see it in a lifetime of practice. In general, the operation is very safe and very successful. Everything depends on the skill of the surgeon, the appropriate choice of procedure and the motivation of the patient. The face-lift, and the ancillary procedures performed with it, represent the only option to undo a lifetime of aging and damage to the face. It seems a shame to consider this when we are now considering strategies to prevent the

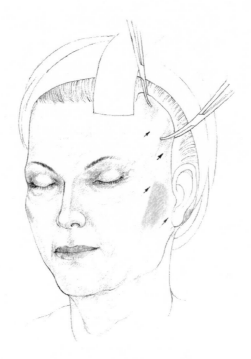

Direction of "lift," in face-lift.

need for it. Here the benefits of starting a program early are out of the reach of mature individuals, but intervention at the earliest reasonable point resets the clock, and saves many good years.

Fees are in the $7,000 to $10,000 range.

[SOMEONE ELSE'S PROBLEMS]

Now the time has come to put all this information to actual use. Before you seek your own place in the scheme, let us share a few examples, and remember, this is the whole regime, not just an invitation to Retin-A or a face-lift.

VICTORIA

Victoria, is a thirty-two-year-old woman. She was married for several years, has no children, currently lives in the Northeast, and works in the financial services industry. Her ancestry is English and German; she has fair skin and light brown hair; she is five feet, six inches tall and weighs 120 pounds. Victoria leads an active life. She skis, plays tennis, and attends an aerobics class three times a week. Although she believes she still looks young, she has recently noticed a few smile lines around her eyes, which don't quite disappear when the smile does. The vertical lines between her eyebrows seem deeper after each day's work, though they are less noticeable when she has a tan.

Victoria is concerned with the changes in her appearance and is determined to take appropriate steps to control matters before they steal her youth.

The Prescription

For a young, fair-skinned woman, sun exposure is a costly indulgence. Victoria is seeing the first signs of heritage, lifestyle, and time and is in transition between requiring prevention and treatment. Here the Youth Corridor program will undo the signs of aging and establish a preventative routine.

Treatment. Several small procedures are necessary to return to ground zero. The most severe complaint is of the increasingly deep vertical lines between the eyebrows. These will be reversed through small incisions in the natural fold of the upper eyelids, beneath the frown lines. Through these half-inch incisions, the corrugator muscles will be divided. That will weaken the ability to create furrows in this area and smooth the brow. The existing line caused by the furrow will be further reduced by fat transplants. The laser resurfacing technique will be applied to alleviating the smile lines, or crow's feet, developing on the cheeks alongside Victoria's eyes.

Additional treatments are directed toward undoing the accumulated sun damage to both the skin surface and deeper layers. For this a series of six concentrated alpha hydroxy acid treatments will be used, two weeks apart and after pretreatment with Retin-A. It will serve to smooth the skin surface, and reduce fine wrinkles, blotches, and scaly areas. The collagen-enhancing qualities of the Retin-A and the AHA will help undo the accumulated sun damage to the elastin and collagen layer of the dermis. That should provide long-term benefit in elasticity and integrity of the skin.

Maintenance

Exercise. Beyond thirty years of age, and with even the earliest loss of elasticity, high-impact aerobics should be discontinued. Substitute a low-impact aerobics program, bicycling, or swimming. All sports should be continued. Outdoor activities, especially water sports, tennis, golf, swimming, and especially skiing, require sunscreen pretreatment. Waterproof and water-resistant varieties are especially valuable in very active individuals, and in this case, must be used.

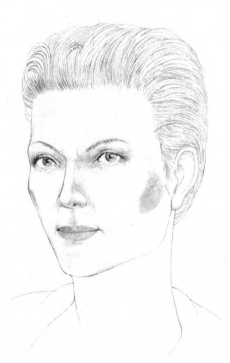

Victoria has frown lines between her eyes and early smile lines.

Nutrition. Since there have been no great weight changes, she is obviously aware of her personal caloric balance. Assuming that this is achieved with an appropriate, healthy diet, few supplements are required. Fruits, vegetables, whole grains, and complex carbohydrates should form the backbone of this diet, but protein and unsaturated fat should be included.

Supplements. Daily: vitamin C, at least 1,000 milligrams; vitamin E, 800 IU.

Evidence for the effectiveness of these antioxidants continues to accumulate. Systemic and specific skin benefits are best derived from dietary supplements. There is no evidence that local application has any value.

Skin care. A fair-skinned individual reporting scaly areas and early wrinkles has dry skin. Moisturization must be vigorous. Moisturizers containing sunscreens are encouraged for daily usage. Soap and water is important at least once daily, particularly when dealing with numerous additives as Victoria must. Her fair skin, so elegant in the past, now is most at risk for early aging. If she wishes to postpone or avoid future cosmetic surgery, Victoria has to make the entire regime a part of her daily life. The routine described begins after the course of Retin-A and AHA has been completed and the skin is no longer irritated.

> **Morning. Gentle soap-and-water wash, followed by refreshing water rinse and application of moisturizer with skin still damp. Moisturizer with sunscreen as a daily habit is preferable if the consistency is pleasant and the product well tolerated. Stinging or irritation are invitations to try another product. Makeup may be applied as usual. Cosmetics containing sunscreen are not nearly as effective, and are not a substitute.**
>
> **Evening. Wash with mild soap and water and rinse. Warm then cold. Same wash routine as in morning. Apply moisture cream containing 2 percent to 8 percent AHA, or use separate products. AHA cream first, then moisture cream. Continue this routine nightly. So long as skin is not irritated,**

there is no need to discontinue treatment. After first three months' usage, continue routine for three weeks each month. Fourth week, substitute non-AHA moisture cream. Resume routine following month. Three on, one off, every month, all year.

Treatment. For a six-month period, every other year, tretinoin treatment should be used nightly. This is applied to the entire face, including previously treated areas of smile lines and lower eyelids. Treatment requires use of sunblock, which is already part of the daily routine. On alternate years, substitute for the tretinoin therapy a series of concentrated, medically supervised AHA peels. These treatments are aimed at retarding further changes in the skin surface and maintaining a smooth surface, free of irregularities and discoloration, and will augment the nightly use of dilute AHA. The routine, plus the treatment schedule, will provide excellent maintenance for a period of five years, at which time the normal changes of aging should be reevaluated, the routine altered, and new treatments offered as appropriate. For this purpose a plastic surgeon or dermatologist familiar with the individual, and willing to offer advice, when indicated, should be consulted. Remember, each routine is directed at current conditions. Conditions change; so must the routine.

Summary. This is the case of an active, young woman, with a genetic predisposition to early aging, who has accelerated the process by sun exposure. She has already seen the first hint of things to come in the form of deepening smile lines, vertical frown lines and irregularities of the skin surface. The treatment and maintenance program outlined is specifically designed to eliminate present damage, maintain what exists, and prevent further accelerating the process. A woman entering the maintenance loop at this point will achieve dramatically positive results of the most subtle and gradual nature. That, after all, is what we are seeking.

The greatest benefit will accrue to those who learn to avoid destructive behavior, and intercept aging early and aggressively. Simply living with natural, unaccelerated aging would be a great step forward for most; actually doing something to modify the changes, a great plus; and actually influencing the process itself, a benefit unheard-of ten years ago. We cannot stop the clock. But we can certainly reset it.

PATRICIA

Patricia is forty-seven years old. She has lived her entire life in sunny southern California. Throughout high school and college and during her early working years, Patricia spent every moment she could at the beach. Her Mediterranean coloration allowed for quick tanning, without the painful sunburns her friends had to endure. Her skin had been slightly oily as a teenager, but she was never bothered with acne. In the twenty-five years since college, she has raised two children, returned to work as an advertising copywriter, gained and lost twenty pounds almost every year, and begun exercising; she uses sunscreen when she remembers to, and has had very little time to devote to herself. Lately, it all seemed to begin to fall apart. Though happily still mostly wrinkle-free, Patricia has noticed vertical lines in her upper lip, which are more noticeable with lipstick. She has become a bit jowly and there is even a hint of a double chin, not fat but loose skin. Previously, all this disappeared when she got down to her fighting weight. This time, she has kept most of the weight off; it's just that the skin hasn't shrunk as it always did in the past. For the first time Patricia is beginning to see her face change, and she doesn't like it.

The Prescription

Patricia has been blessed with thick, moist skin that responds to the sun with immediate tanning. This enhanced pigment further protects the skin from burning. Unfortunately, it does not prevent the accelerated disruption of elastin and collagen fibers caused by ultraviolet rays. The loss of elasticity and loosening of facial skin has been markedly hastened by the sun. Ten to twenty cigarettes a day have also taken their toll. Although her skin type has thus far protected her from damage in the form of fine wrinkles, the actual act of smoking cigarettes, the repetitive lip-pursing motion, has folded the vertical lines into her lips. It is not unusual for the upper lip to be worse than the lower, but both soon become pleated and the lines accentuated by runs of lipstick. What must take place here is reeducation, repair, and renewal. The loose skin of the jowls and under the chin area is ideally sited for a layered S-lift. Before any surgery can be performed, the patient must stop smoking for six weeks. Blood vessel constriction resulting from smoking cigarettes creates a unique risk of skin damage and scarring at surgery. The side benefit after surgery is that continued abstinence promotes better blood supply and healthier skin. Patricia has the excess upper-eyelid skin so frequently

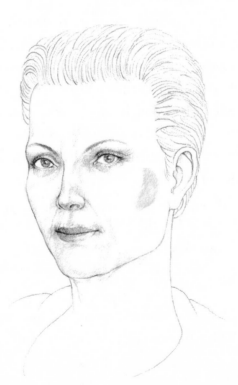

Patricia has vertical lines on her upper lip and some loose skin.

present at this stage, which, with any lower-eyelid problems, will be dealt with at the same time. The lip lines are dealt with by laser resurfacing performed at the same time. The absence of fine wrinkling precludes the need for skin peel, which would involve significant risk of discoloration in one with dark skin and a history of prolonged sun exposure. Laser facial resurfacing appears to present less risk of discoloration and should be considered when fine wrinkling is a problem. It is not a consideration in this case. She will begin a six-month course of tretinoin and must become devoted to the use of sunscreen. If Patricia is unable, or unwilling, to use sunscreens, the tretinoin therapy is precluded. This is an example of the need for the patient to help herself. There is every reason to believe the tretinoin therapy will undo some of the sun damage, but it is imperative to use sunscreen during and after treatment to avoid discoloration, and of course, to prevent further damage.

These procedures will undo most of the grossly visible damage, and leave Patricia with clean facial angles, skin that fits, and relatively free of lip lines.

Maintenance

Exercise. Patricia has managed to control her weight. She has stopped smoking as a preoperative precaution, and must not resume. The withdrawal will cause a nervous need for replacement. That usually takes the form of binge eating. This is a perfect time to substitute exercise, a far more gratifying and less dangerous habit. A structured program may require some professional guidance at the start, and becomes a passion as results are seen. This will curb appetite by several means including fatigue, substitution, and an unwillingness to undo the good one has worked so hard to achieve. The program should include significant aerobic exercise in the form of walking, bicycling, and best of all, swimming. Muscle building and tone maintenance are crucial for a forty-seven-year-old woman who has not been exercising regularly and well. This means weight training as well as aerobics. Osteoporosis and shrinking muscle mass are prevalent in nonexercising women after menopause. It seems far more reasonable to be in good shape earlier, and face the hormonal changes and their side effects stronger and healthier. There is considerable evidence that much older individuals, men and women alike, in their seventies and beyond, are able to build muscle and increase range of motion and bone density with regular exercise. It is never too late to get in shape, and surely never too early.

Nutrition. Patricia is most definitely not in control of her nutrition. That she routinely gains ten or twenty pounds is proof enough, though her ability to keep it off this time is a strongly positive sign. This speaks for commitment. Maintenance will be aided by the tips on page 30. Additionally, Patricia should sharply reduce the fat in her diet. This is most easily done by reducing the amount of animal fat in the diet. Elimination of beef and chicken is not necessary. But chicken skin, which is where the fat is stored, should be eliminated, and beef should be limited to once a week. Butter and eggs should be curtailed to the point of elimination, and fried foods are out altogether. These guidelines are not intentionally heart-smart, but limiting fat creates by far the healthiest diet. For Patricia's purposes the fat restrictions are based on the simple fact that fat contains more than twice the calories as an equivalent amount of carbohydrate or protein. This simple dietary change will not force her to become a vegetarian. It requires little sacrifice. The number of calories consumed is halved. She will be better able to maintain her optimal weight, and who knows, she may just live longer.

Supplements. Daily: vitamin C, 1,000 milligrams; vitamin E, 800 IU.
Consider estrogen replacement as natural menopause approaches. Early replacement as levels dip may serve to help ward off early skin changes.

Skin care routine. Patricia needs to find ground zero in her routine. The copious oil production of youth has declined, though areas such as her nose and forehead tend to glisten as the day wears on. She has little need for moisturizers.

In fact, she still possesses the best moisturizer of all, her own lubricating oils. Well-balanced and proper for her skin, there is no problem with allergy or irritation. Some people, though not Patricia, actually react to their own skin oils. This condition is a form of seborrhea, and is one of the few conditions in which one's own oils are not the best choice. Patricia must wash with soap and water at least twice daily. The warm/cold routine is best. After washing she must remember sunscreen. That is imperative in a sunny southwestern climate. Each application of soap removes most of the sunscreen, so it must be replenished. If there is an oil buildup on the nose or forehead, repeated washing is permissible. This happens often in warm climates with moderate humidity. The oil level of the rest of the face may need an occasional boost, but this will be the exception, not the rule.

Daily (day or night application). AHA cream should be a part of the regular routine. That may help undo some of the collagen and elastin damage caused by sun exposure, and will keep the skin surface smooth and blemish-free.

Summary. Patricia is the sort of individual who will find the greatest improvement from surgical tightening of the loose skin, and laser resurfacing of her lip lines. She is otherwise blessed with healthy, moist, unlined skin, and needs lifestyle reeducation to avoid making matters worse at a time in her life when they might not be so easily corrected. At this point her appearance will be remarkably youthful for forty-seven, and should stay that way for the next fifteen years.

ELLEN

Ellen is twenty-three years old. She has just moved to Los Angeles, from her home in Florida, for a role in a television series. For the previous four years, she was a model and is very aware of her appearance, for both professional and personal reasons. She is thin, thin, fair-skinned, athletic, and very attractive. Best of all, the camera loves her, and accentuates her high cheekbones and angular face.

Ellen inherited these features from her Scandinavian mother, and shares them with most of the extended family. Unfortunately, she has seen her mother age "overnight," and look like an old woman before she was fifty. With this example, and an awareness of the dangers of Miami sunshine, Ellen is religious about protecting her skin. She is young and still looks wonderful, but is interested in doing all she can to prevent the rapid aging her mother underwent. She has no specific complaints.

The Prescription

This young woman is seeking a routine at the right time. Before there is damage. She has suffered little ultraviolet damage and is aware of the effects of unharnessed facial aging in her family.

Treatment. No specific treatments or surgical intervention of any sort are indicated. This situation requires education and prevention, and offers the opportunity to maintain a healthy youthful appearance for the next thirty years and beyond.

Maintenance

Exercise. Encouraging exercise in this case is unnecessary. Ellen swims, works out, and plays squash. All excellent activities. She should be counseled against more than the occasional running she does on weekends, and encouraged to use low-impact aerobic activities such as distance swimming and cycling as substitutes. Ellen's generation understands the value of exercise. She is well-advised to make time for a daily routine even as she assumes the rigorous schedule of early calls for work.

Nutrition. This is a problem. Ellen must be thin for her career, and has inflicted strict dietary rules upon herself. So rigid is she that meals are sacrificed and a full, balanced diet is virtually impossible. Obviously, she has enough caloric intake to meet the demands of a busy professional life and fuel her athletic activities as well. Therefore, little more than advice on incorporating important nutrients is indicated. All this will likely change with age. But since she avoids fat and empty calories, and takes vitamin supplements, nothing need be addressed at present.

Supplements. In addition to the multivitamins and numerous fad additives to which Ellen periodically subscribes, she is encouraged to add antioxidants to the routine. Daily: vitamin C, at least 1,000 milligrams; vitamin E, 800 IU.

These antioxidants may be skin specific, and evidence for their general effectiveness continues to accumulate.

Skin care. Ellen has fair skin that she has protected from the sun since childhood. She is quite expert in the use of cosmetics, and removes them with industrial-strength cleansers. She has shunned the use of simple soap and water since entering the profession, and has spent the majority of working days covered in various forms of stage makeup. She has a special need to find ground zero and treat her skin sensibly. That includes the removal of makeup with whatever cleansers work, followed by soap and water and vigorous towel drying. The thorough soap-and-water cleansing routine is followed twice daily, morning and night. When makeup removal is necessary after the workday and before evening, a third thorough soap-and-water wash is indicated. Each is followed by application of moisturizer. The morning routine is by moisturizer containing sunblock. This is an important step to remember in sunny climates. The incidental sun exposure has a cumulative effect, and should be protected against. After moisturizer, makeup can be applied. Ellen understands good skin care and protection, but must take care to fully clear her skin of makeup and denatured oils and remoisturize.

Daily (day or night application). AHA cream should become part of the regular routine. It is applied before moisturizer or in a combination product with moisturizer. The low-acid concentration will serve as a daily exfoliant, particularly important in someone whose skin surface is contaminated with layers of foreign substances. The AHA will also help keep the skin surface smooth, even in color, and blemish-free and seems to help undo whatever collagen damage has been incurred. This should be used daily for three weeks, then stopped for one week each month.

Summary. Ellen needs no treatment. An intelligent preventative routine will help keep her beautiful into middle age. Though sun damage may be minimal, and not readily visible, it very likely exists. A six-month course of tretinoin could aid in reversing this collagen damage, and should be considered in the next several years.

This is the sort of individual who with minimal sun exposure as a child can enter the program early, and grow gracefully ageless with it.

individual checklist for skin care and

MAINTENANCE ROUTINE

Facial changes over the years are generally quite predictable. Individual variation does occur and is usually related to genetic skin type and lifestyle. Understand that the inexorable course of events affects all of us in our own special way, but leaves none of us untouched. If some aspect of facial aging is more rapid in your mirror than your neighbors', then find solace in the fact that the pace and the place may vary, but no one is immune. Rather than take issue with the calendar of changes, understand them to be the general scheme of things. In many specifics, you will find yourself ahead of or behind the calendar. Whatever the case, you will find much of yourself here. And if you find the course compelling in its accuracy, be consoled in the realization that there is something you can do about it.

Here is how this section works. The individual checklist is fairly difficult to face. It offers nothing complimentary other than unchecked lines, representing problems you don't have. Otherwise it is your own reality check. It will help establish your position and identify problems that must be accepted, or dealt with. All the *symptoms* can be dealt with, and the solutions are not necessarily onerous or frightening. The earlier one considers dealing with these issues, the less there will be to deal with. Even at later stages of life, one need not feel compelled to rush off for cosmetic surgery. That is not the purpose of this program. Resetting the clock may not be the goal for everyone. Nonetheless, all can benefit from the simple, age-related programs described here. It takes little effort to avoid making things worse, and not much more to help things along. Establish your situation on the checklist. Then read through the age-specific guide. This is organized at five-year intervals, and represents average status. Use that as your guide. If you don't fit into your age group, congratulations. Read a notch younger and count your blessings. Some will find themselves ahead of the curve. It isn't the end of the world. Again, you are not a prisoner of these changes. There is something you can do about each and every one of them, but first, you must see the pattern clearly, then determine its importance in your life.

I do not believe that a desperate attempt to correct each sign of facial aging is appropriate. Surely the reality of all this is difficult enough to take, without enduring the philosophy of a plastic surgeon. But having lived in this odd little circumscribed environment for more than two decades, certain truths become apparent to me. The ultimate goal of this exercise should be to look as good on the outside as you feel on the inside. And indeed, looking good will make you feel better as well. Our goal is to age slowly and gracefully, and to avoid accelerating the process by destructive behavior. I applaud any attempt to skew the curve and visibly retard aging, but the result must look natural. Relentless pursuit of youth, unmodified by common sense, becomes a caricature, and by its own nature, is self-defeating. There is little excuse for such behavior. Nor does there appear to be common sense in aggravating the aging process by refusing to unlearn bad habits, or refusing to make small efforts for rich dividends in a healthy and attractive appearance.

The following information is organized to include cosmetic surgery, nonsurgical treatments, and self-care. Even if you elect not to consider the treatment or surgical options, you will still benefit from adopting the skin care routine alone. Read on, choose what you like, but be certain to consider the information. Each time you put off applying yourself is a day lost, whatever your age.

Checklist

- Circles under eyes
- Fine wrinkles under eyes
- Smile lines outside eyes
- Dry or blotchy skin
- Oily, irregular skin
- Discoloration or abnormal pigment
- Deepening nasolabial line or fold
- Nasolabial line etched into skin
- Parentheses lines at corners of mouth
- Vertical frown lines between eyebrows
- Vertical lines on upper lip
- Fine wrinkles on cheeks
- Slight fullness along jawline; loss of clean line
- Fullness under jawline
- Small fatty pouches alongside mouth
- Irregular patches of color on skin

The previous simple problems can be easily corrected without surgery. Some require biochemical skin treatments, some microsuction. The following portion of the checklist can only be effectively dealt with surgically.

- Excess skin of eyelids
- Puffiness under eyes
- Nasolabial folds fully developed and line etched into skin
- Vertical lines between eyebrows deepening
- Jowls develop over jawline
- Hanging skin and deep facial wrinkles
- Loss of cheekbone fullness; drooping cheeks

Check off descriptions that pertain to you. For the most part, they will form a cluster about your age group. The methods for dealing with the various problems have all been discussed in the chapters on skin care, over-the-counter preparations, medical treatments, and surgery. The personal programs begin with age twenty-five. Although certain routines would be well begun earlier, there is so much variation in skin condition at this point, and little need for generalized care, that few simple recommendations will be made for the youngest concerned individuals. From age twenty-five forward, the program will change in five-year increments. *Remember:* The age-grouped symptoms are only generalizations. They do not pertain to everyone. Find the changes that best reflect your situation and proceed from there.

[ALL AGES UNDER TWENTY-FIVE]

Wash twice daily with soap and water. Warm wash, then cold rinse. Towel dry.

Use sunscreen during all outdoor activities: SPF 15 or greater. Use water-resistant or waterproof sunscreen for swimming. Suntan creams and oils are *not* sunscreens, and offer no protection.

All other skin care should be related to specific problems, and should be discussed with your dermatologist.

[TWENTY-FIVE]

Conditions. Skin characteristics will be virtually unchanged from adolescence, except for a decreasing susceptibility to acnelike eruptions. These require a dermatologist's care. Skin may become slightly drier. No visible changes in the form

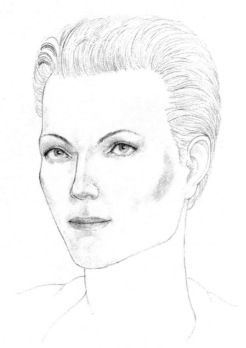

Twenty-five:
No visible changes, though biochemical denaturing of collagen has begun.

of wrinkles or lines, but irregularities of the surface and slight discolorations may be present. In the dermis, collagen and elastin, which provide the resilience of the skin, are already damaged, though no outward signs can yet be seen.

Nutrition. This is the time in life to begin weight stabilization. Growth and teenage hormones are under control, and there should be little variation in weight going forward to middle age. The value of low fat intake and increased fruit and vegetable intake must become a habit from this point. There is nothing wrong with eating a steak, but that should become the exception not the rule.

Supplements. Daily: vitamin C, 1,000 milligrams; vitamin E, 800 IU.

Exercise. Exercise should be vigorous, both at sport and for conditioning. Aerobic activity can be unrestricted. Attempt to adopt a low-impact program. Regular, every-other-day workout routine includes aerobic activity and weight training.

Skin care routine.

1. **Wash face twice daily with soap and water. Warm wash then cold rinse. Towel dry. If skin is dry, wash with soap, then moisturize. If skin is oily, wash with soap and do not moisturize.**
2. **Moisturize as necessary, particularly during winter months and reduced humidity. Daily use of moisturizer with sunscreen is encouraged; it should be applied every morning.**
3. **Use sunscreens of SPF 15 or greater during all outdoor activities; water-resistant or waterproof sunscreen for swimming.**
4. **Nightly, on alternating weeks, apply AHA cream after washing. Then apply moisturizer.**

[THIRTY]

Conditions. The first signs of smile lines appear at the corners of the eyes. Lower lids show a few lines below the lashes. An upper-eyelid fold of skin is visible when eyes open, but with little or no overhang. Skin condition is slightly drier. As at age twenty-five, there are significant, but no longer unseen, changes taking place within the collagen and elastin of the dermis. These are first demonstrated at this point as the fine lines around the eyes.

Nutrition. This is a particularly important period in which positive habits and routines must be learned. Job stress, sex, marriage, and childbirth compete for time and attention during these years. Weight change, frequently weight gain, often appears. Weight optimization and stabilization are more easily learned here than later. Adequate and varied diet based primarily on fruits, vegetables, and complex carbohydrates is necessary for the above reasons as well as for provision of naturally occurring antioxidants and avoidance of detrimental food groups.

Supplements. Daily: vitamin C, 1,000 milligrams; vitamin E, 800 IU.

Exercise. Vigorous activities and all sports are encouraged. Avoid all high-impact aerobic activities. Swim, fast-walk, bike. Curtail distance running. Weight training for muscle tone.

Skin care routine.

1. **Wash face twice daily with soap and water. Towel dry.**
2. **Moisturize daily. Apply sunscreen daily. Moisturizer containing sunscreen can be used.**
3. **Nightly: Wash with soap and water. Apply AHA cream nightly three weeks out of four for six months. After a full six-month regime, switch to tretinoin (Retin-A) for the next six months. Alternate through the five-year period, or until changes are seen in the skin.**

Tretinoin is applied to clean, dry skin nightly. It may be irritating at first. This is usually self-limited and is usually relieved by moisturizer application. Sunscreen must be applied regularly during this period. The use of tretinoin is intended to prevent and combat disruptive changes within the collagen layer. This is nonspecific and should be applied to all exposed areas of the face and neck. Specific areas are treated as well. They will most likely be the fine skin around the eyes where the first wrinkles are becoming noticeable. The application of tretinoin in these areas requires no greater attention or dosage than the remainder of the facial skin, just don't forget them.

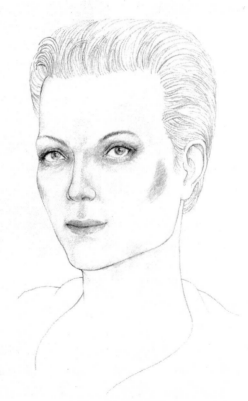

Thirty–thirty-five:
Fine lines around eyes and early nasolabial fold.

4. Sunscreen of SPF 15 or greater during all outdoor activities. This is particularly important once tretinoin use has begun.

Procedures. These are usually not yet necessary. Toward the end of this period, as the individual approaches thirty-five, there are the first changes requiring the consideration of intervention. For most, these will be centered about the eyelids. With the institution of good care in the form of tretinoin and AHA creams, the need for intervention will be pushed back.

[THIRTY-FIVE]

Conditions. Skin will become drier than in the past. Smile lines about the eyes will be noticeable. Nasolabial lines will deepen and approach the corners of the mouth. For many, vertical frown lines between the eyebrows will deepen. Excess skin of the upper eyelids will appear to varying degrees and the lower-lid area will become puffier more often. Though there is little significant loosening of the skin, damage to collagen and elastin will have occurred and fullness may be developing in the lower face. This represents early loss of elasticity.

In general, these changes will be manifested to some degree during the period from thirty-five to forty. The changes, when they occur, are in the early stages, and though not terribly detracting from youthful good looks, are a sign of a different stage in life.

Nutrition. As discussed previously, this period continues to be the most physically demanding. Professional responsibilities, childbearing and raising necessities, and a wealth of physical demands accrue. It is a particularly important period during which to maintain control. There are so many reasons and excuses for forgetting about nutrition and exercise for a while, and getting on with the important things in life, that we lose sight of the fact that these are among the important things in life. Good nutrition should have become a part of your life

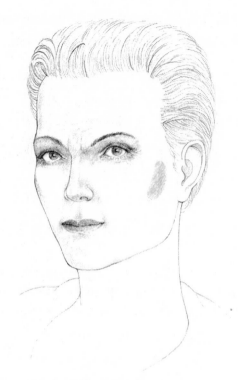

Thirty-five–forty:
Smile lines, deepening nasolabial fold, vertical frown lines, and some excess eyelid skin.

by now. A salad and fresh fruit are as easily accessible as cookies and ice cream, and not only are they far better for you, they also set a good example. Perhaps your family won't have to unlearn dietary tastes as we had to. With fewer calories being spent on physical activities, caloric intake should be carefully controlled. For most women, this becomes a period when dietary extremes take over. Neither denial nor indulgence is acceptable, though viewed from the perspective of facial aging, more damage is done by excessive weight, which stretches and breaks down elastic fibers, than by being too thin, which if not carried to anorexia, only results in an unattractive appearance, and can easily be corrected with weight gain. In any event, thirty-five to forty is not the time to experiment.

Once again: low calorie intake; low-fat, high-complex-carbohydrate diets, with adequate protein. Limit the amount of protein from animal sources. Fresh fruit and vegetables should make up as large a portion of calorie intake as possible.

Supplements. Daily: vitamin C, 1,000 milligrams; vitamin E, 800 IU.

Exercise. Although it becomes increasingly difficult to participate, physical activities are crucial. This is the time to maintain conditioning and fitness. What is lost here becomes increasingly difficult to regain.

Running, other than short-distance warm-up, should be abandoned in favor of any other aerobic workout. Bicycling, fast walking, and swimming are encouraged. StairMaster and rowing machines, among other devices, provide good aerobic workouts, but are dependent on availability and physical condition. Simply walking briskly for twenty minutes per day provides enough aerobic activity for cardiac protection, but that is not enough activity for age thirty-five. Active sports and weight training are advised. Two 45-minute workouts per week will maintain muscle tone. Three will build muscle and strength. Don't worry about becoming a "muscle girl"; this won't do it.

Skin care routine.

1. **Wash face twice daily with mild soap and water. Warm wash then cold rinse.**

2. **Apply AHA cream or lotion, or moisturizing lotion containing AHA each morning. Then apply sunscreen and makeup as usual. The addition of AHA to the morning routine should not cause visible irritation or be noticeable.**

3. **Nightly, wash and towel dry. Apply tretinoin to areas of visible wrinkles nightly, then moisturize.**

4. **For six months each year, apply tretinoin cream to entire face, including areas already being treated. This is applied as a general aid to the collagen and elastin fibers of the dermis, and is not aimed at specific tar-**

gets. The tretinoin cream is used in the evenings, the AHA in the morning.

5. Sunscreens are a must. Morning application should be supplemented during outdoor activities.

Procedures. Microsuction for early fullness at the jawline or cheeks, and for nasolabial folds, yields immediate relief, and also slows future changes.

Smile lines and lower-eyelid wrinkles are pretreated with tretinoin and peeled with trichloroacetic acid. That is usually adequate when begun early. Later stages are best treated with laser resurfacing.

Puffiness of lower lids is treated with subconjunctival blepharoplasty and peels.

[FORTY]

Conditions. The transition from thirty-five to forty is less dramatic physically than emotionally, for while one may consider this a milestone of maturity, the aging process continues quietly and inexorably forward. Changes that began several years ago slowly amplify. Nasolabial folds deepen. Eyelid skin loosens. Wrinkles around eyes deepen if not previously treated. There is a slight loosening of skin at the jawline and below, with fat accumulation. Fine wrinkles and blemishes are particularly evident on fair-skinned individuals. Verti-cal lines between eyebrows deepen. Early vertical lines may be noted on the upper lip.

Nutrition. Unabated physical demands accompany early hormonal changes. Diet based on grains, complex carbohydrates, fruits, and vegetables will provide all the elements of good nutrition. Caloric intake is more easily controlled with this sort of diet. Fat restriction begun earlier now becomes doubly important as estrogen levels deplete over this decade. Nutritional habits begun earlier are important for all aspects of overall health.

Supplements. Daily: vitamin C, 1,000 milligrams; vitamin E, 800 IU.

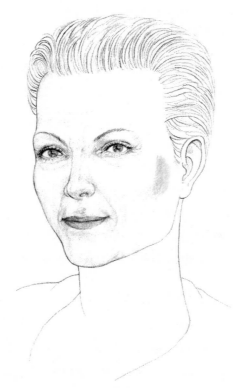

Forty–forty-five:
Changes accelerate.

Exercise. Active sports become less important as a source of aerobic conditioning, and must be replaced by strict exercise programs. These must include impact-free aerobics, and range-of-motion and strength training. Routines must be performed at least three times weekly to meet goals. Twenty minutes of walking, swimming, rowing, or bicycling can be performed as often as daily. Weight and range-of-motion training as often as daily, and as infrequently as three times weekly.

If strength-building routines are done daily, muscle groups exercised should be alternated. Muscles need a day of rest to recover from vigorous exercise. If the exercise performed has not been vigorous and strenuous, its value has been diminished. Whenever possible, it is best to establish exercise routines with a qualified physical fitness trainer.

Skin care routine.

1. Wash twice daily with soap and water. Warm wash, cold rinse, then towel dry.
2. Apply moisturizer daily, and AHA daily for three weeks of four.
3. Nightly: Apply tretinoin cream to entire face for six months each year. It is applied as a general aid to the collagen and elastin fibers of the dermis, as well as a direct treatment to combat fine wrinkles developing in the facial skin. It works well with the morning use of AHA cream.
4. Apply Tretinoin cream to trouble spots such as smile lines and lip lines during the six-month rest period for the remainder of facial skin. AHA cream is continued each morning throughout.
5. Sunscreen must be used daily. This is particularly crucial to avoid discoloration from tretinoin and sunlight. If one wishes the benefits of tretinoin therapy, one must use sunscreen at all times of exposure. This provides double benefit in the form of the tretinoin effect and protection from the damaging effect of the sun in general and the problems that would be caused by sun exposure to tretinoin treated skin.

Procedures. A series of professional concentration AHA peels are augmented by the daily application of low-concentration AHA cream, as described above. Collagen, or fat transplants, is employed for deeper facial lines; blepharoplasty, to correct excess skin of the upper eyelids and puffy skin and wrinkles of the lower lids. This is often accompanied by a TCA peel of the lower-lid skin, which does much to reverse fine wrinkling and discoloration. At the time of blepharoplasty, or as an isolated procedure, the corrugator muscles are resected to combat vertical frown lines between eyebrows. Existing furrows may be treated with collagen or fat transplants to correct depth. Microsuction of the jawline returns a clean line, tightens skin, and slows further changes. Microsuction of nasolabial lines reduces depth. Laser resurfacing erases the vertical lines of upper lip.

[FORTY-FIVE]

Conditions. The last five years of this decade from forty to fifty witness the loss of the battle with gravity. Differing vastly among individuals, the process cannot be denied. Collagen and elastin denature, stretch, and break, accelerated by lifestyle in most cases, and more slowly by natural attrition in others. Whatever the circumstances and extent, there is loosening of the skin. Nasolabial lines become cheek folds. Pockets of fat may develop outside the mouth. The corners of the mouth begin to look downward due to loose tissue above, and folds and fat alongside. Cheekbones become masked as subcutaneous padding drops below the prominence. The skin of the neck no longer bounces back from stretching, and a slight excess develops. Vertical lines deepen on the upper lip. Smile lines deepen, as do frown lines, and eyelid skin shows excess and overhang. Fine wrinkles more pronounced on cheeks become deeper.

The skin about the upper eyelids has stretched and become redundant, sometimes actually resting on the lashes. Puffiness and wrinkles mar the lower lids. Deep frown lines have set between the eyebrows. These changes will have become evident years earlier, and should have been dealt with at the time the manifestations appeared. We shall mention them now to complete an accurate survey of expected changes at this stage.

To a greater or lesser degree, all these things happen. Within the next five years, they will accelerate and demand attention for the majority of people. Twenty years of maintenance, if it had been available, would have done much to prevent, hold back, and mask these changes. Unfortunately, we have only recently come upon both the tools and the organization to help lead more gracefully into this period. Changes noted in the previous five-year period, to age forty-five, will be addressed again. Years of AHA, tretinoin, sunscreen, and good habits would likely have had a major positive effect on maintaining the integrity of collagen and elastin, and therefore significantly retarded the appearance of laxity and wrinkles.

Nutrition. The years from forty-five to fifty see many metabolic changes. Calorie needs are reduced. Subcutaneous fat seems to be undergoing redistribu-

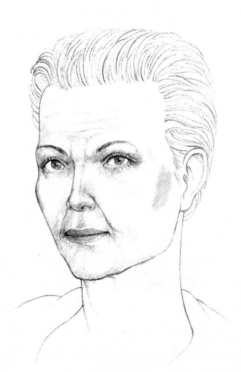

Forty-five–fifty:
Changes continue. Loss of elasticity becomes noticeable.

tion and gaining on us. Childbearing years end and many enter natural menopause. Physical activities consume less of one's schedule and lack of exercise takes a toll.

Calorie intake must be closely related to needs. Weight gain at this juncture would result in irreversible stretching of skin. The fact that individuals at this stage of life often find themselves unable to digest heavy meals taken in the evening is an undeniable indication that the digestive and metabolic processes have changed. Just as one's needs diminish with changes in bodily function, so does the physiological ability to tolerate the intake necessary in the building years. Light meals, less protein, more fruit and vegetables, more water, and much less fat are called for.

Supplements. Daily: vitamin C, 1,000 milligrams; vitamin E, 800 IU. Calcium supplement, either as calcium tablets or in multivitamins.

Exercise. Force yourself. This is a very important period. Exercise should be vigorous enough to provide aerobic conditioning and muscle building. Good muscle size and strength are closely followed by increased bone density, which is essential in the prevention of osteoporosis and the full enjoyment of a healthy middle life. There should be nothing physically impossible at this point in life except childbearing. For manifold reasons your parents were old at fifty. That is unthinkable today. The first line of defense is physical activity, and this must include conditioning. Working out isn't fun, but do it now and improve the quality of the next thirty years of your life.

Skin care routine.

1. **Wash face twice daily with soap and water. Lather with warm water. Rinse. Repeat, then final rinse with cold water.**
2. **Mornings: After washing, apply AHA cream daily for three weeks of every four. Apply moisturizer, or moisturizer-containing sunscreen, to dampened skin after AHA application.**

3. A sunscreen of SPF 15 or greater should be used daily, with particular attention paid with the use of tretinoin. When spending time outdoors and undergoing tretinoin therapy, sunscreen should be replenished regularly, particularly after swimming or sweating.

4. Nightly, after washing and carefully drying skin, apply tretinoin cream in a thin layer to clean, dry skin. Follow with moisturizer. Do this every night as long as skin does not become irritated. The effects of tretinoin are cumulative and need several months to become established. Use nightly for five months of every six.

Treatments.

1. Tretinoin cream nightly as above.
2. Yearly medical-concentration alpha hydroxy acid peel series to maintain smooth, regular skin surface and control fine wrinkles and blemishes.

Procedures. Here we must assume that though they may have been suggested, no procedures have been performed to this point.

The loss of laxity varies greatly from individual to individual at this fairly early stage. Later, there will be changes enough in virtually everyone to warrant attention. Here one must recognize what is happening and compare the changes with one's personal standards. A layered S-lift is the ideal mechanism to correct facial laxity at this stage. It is performed in conjunction with micro-suction of the jawline, jowls, and under the chin, as well as along the nasolabial folds and the fat pockets beside the corners of the mouth. Upper- and lower-lid blepharoplasty are performed at the same time, if they haven't been done before. Corrugator muscles are resected through the upper-lid incision if vertical frown lines are a problem. If possible, the skin is prepared with AHA treatments prior to surgery, and a deep peel may be performed if wrinkling of the cheeks persists. Deep smile lines and vertical lines of the upper lip are treated with the CO_2 laser.

It is unusual for women forty-five to fifty years old to need full face-lifts and deep peels. Most are still quite youthful looking, and have become aware of the impending loss of the battle with gravity, the sun, and the calendar. Much can be done to restore full youthful good looks at this point, but there are no more shortcuts.

[FIFTY TO FIFTY-FIVE]

Conditions.   This is the big time. There is no disguising it; things have changed, will change before too long, or are even imminent as you look at what is happening to the friends around you. No more fooling around. The ages of fifty to fifty-five affect most women dramatically. Often unnecessarily dramatically. So far there have been no precipitous changes, just the gradual effects of aging and the onset and acceptance of menopause. You are still young and vital. Call it something else, and get on with the business of living.

Nothing happens at fifty that hasn't been creeping up on you for forty-nine years. The changes are gradual, including menopause, which may actually have occurred earlier. Loss of elasticity continues, and the changes described in the previous sections increase arithmetically. There is simply more of the same, and it can be dealt with similarly, if a bit more aggressively.

If no surgery has been done to this point, there will likely be excess skin, and perhaps, hooding of the upper eyelids. The lower lids will be wrinkled and per-

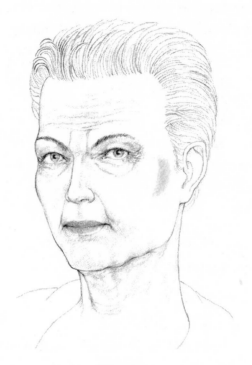

Fifty–sixty:
Loss of elasticity and wrinkling become more profound.

haps puffy. Vertical frown lines between the eyebrows will have deepened, and the eyebrows themselves will have dropped somewhat. Horizontal lines of the forehead deepen. Nasolabial folds deepen and the line becomes etched into the skin. Lines deepen at corners of the mouth, accentuated by small fat pockets. Cheekbones look less prominent as subcutaneous fat padding drops. Early jowls interrupt clean line of jaw, and loose skin becomes evident under the chin. The platysma muscle loosens and forms two vertical bands that appear at the front of the neck. Vertical lines deepen on upper lip and wrinkles are noted on cheeks both from accumulated collagen damage and reduction in circulating estrogen.

Nutrition. Nutritional standards are unchanged from forty-five. Caloric needs have diminished and weight gain seems to result from the slightest indiscretion. Significant weight gain must be avoided, as the skin has lost elasticity and will be permanently stretched. Heavy meals are poorly digested, resulting in a feeling of lassitude, and should be avoided. Fruit, vegetables, grain, and complex carbohydrates should comprise the framework of your diet. It should have less animal protein and much less fat. Reduction in dietary fat reduces calories, as fat contains more than twice the calories of either protein or carbohydrates. At least as important is the fact that after menopause the incidence of heart disease in women skyrockets. This runs a parallel course with the loss of the protective effect of estrogen, and though one may find protection with estrogen supplements, a more alert lifestyle is indicated. Drink at least a quart of clear fluids daily, preferably water. Alcoholic beverages within reason. There have been no large-scale studies that I know of to determine whether alcohol reduces the incidence of heart diseases in postmenopausal women as it does in men, so enjoy it, but use it frugally.

Supplements. Daily: vitamin C, 1,000 milligrams; vitamin E, 800 IU. Calcium supplement, daily. Estrogen replacement as indicated.

Exercise. As active sports activities are reduced, aerobic and muscle training must increase. Aerobic fitness is cardiovascular fitness and is directly related to all forms of physical performance, from golf to sex. It is directly related to longevity and must be maintained.

If one has not worked with a trainer before, this is a great time to begin. Muscle mass and muscle tone are related to maintaining bone density and the prevention of osteoporosis. Exercising must become a habit. Real exercise yields real results. Don't fool yourself. Waving your arms around twice a week is not enough. Work out for an hour at least three times a week. Fast-walking, bicycling, walking a StairMaster, and swimming are excellent aerobic exercises and great warmups for weight training. No running. If you ran before, cut down or stop. If you are not a runner, don't start now.

Not only will serious workouts be crucial for your well-being, you will look better and feel great.

Skin care routine.

1. **Wash twice daily with soap and water. Lather with warm water, rinse, then repeat, then rinse with cold.**
2. **Apply AHA cream after washing in the morning.**
3. **Apply moisturizer or sunscreen with moisturizer after AHA.**
4. **If using separate sunscreen, apply after AHA, then moisturizer.**
5. **If using combination products, sunscreen must be supplemented during the day. Combination AHA, sunscreen, and moisturizer may provide inadequate moisturization. This, too, can be supplemented during the day, and is essential while tretinoin is being used. After menopause there is considerably more troublesome dryness. This should be treated as it occurs. The remedy is water and moisturizer.**
6. **Nightly, apply tretinoin cream after washing and drying face, followed by moisturizer.**

Procedures. During the early fifties, the changes requiring surgery differ only slightly from the previous plateau. The excess skin of the upper eyelids and puffiness and wrinkled skin of the lowers can be corrected by blepharoplasty, if it hasn't been done before. Lower-eyelid skin may also need peel for fine wrinkles and discoloration. Upper-lid incision may be used for corrugator resection when necessary for treatment of vertical frown lines between eyebrows; and microsuction for the jawline, under the chin, nasolabial folds, and fat pockets beside the mouth; Laser or peel for smile lines, vertical lines of the upper lip, and corners of the mouth.

If facial laxity has not progressed beyond the last stage, a layered S-lift will suffice. Most often this is the case. There is no advantage in doing more than is necessary. Toward he middle and end of the decade, wrinkling becomes more severe and the skin of the neck loosens. Reversing this requires a full face-lift, including the lower neck. The two bands in the front of the neck are the leading edges of the now lax platysma muscle, and are tightened through a small incision under the jaw. Peeling or CO_2 laser resurfacing may be necessary in order to reset the clock as effectively as possible.

AFTERWORD
THE YOUTH CORRIDOR

The point constantly underscored throughout this book is that you can maintain an unchanged youthful appearance through the years from thirty to fifty-five or sixty. Can you remain exactly the same? No. But you can remain largely unchanged by the stigmata of aging. The tools are readily available, and you only have one chance. You must avail yourself of them now, and make an effort at self-help.

For those starting young enough, a youthful appearance will be a lifetime gift. For those in the early stages of visible aging, we can turn back the clock and offer a fresh start. For those already in middle age we can offer a dramatic reversal, and the knowledge necessary to slow future aging. There is something here for everyone, at every stage of life, but you must make the effort.

Live smarter.
Live better.
Care for yourself now.
Enjoy your life fully and beautifully.